GESTATIONAL

DIABETES

COOKBOOK

Dietitian approved low sugar and carbs diabetic recipes for its reversal and for prediabetes

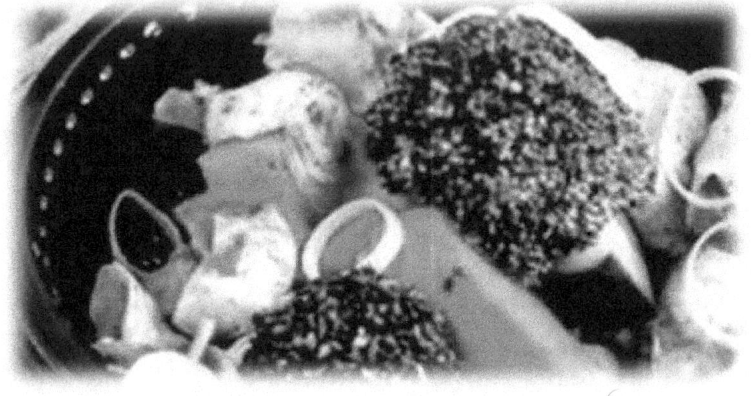

Dr. Grace Hester

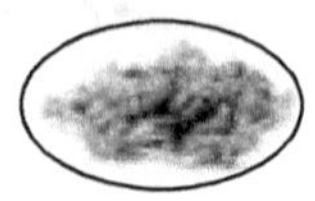 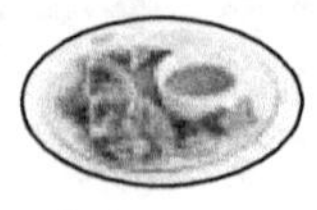 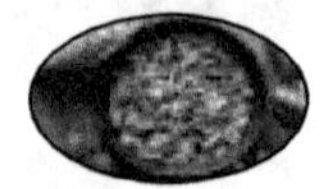

Copyright Page

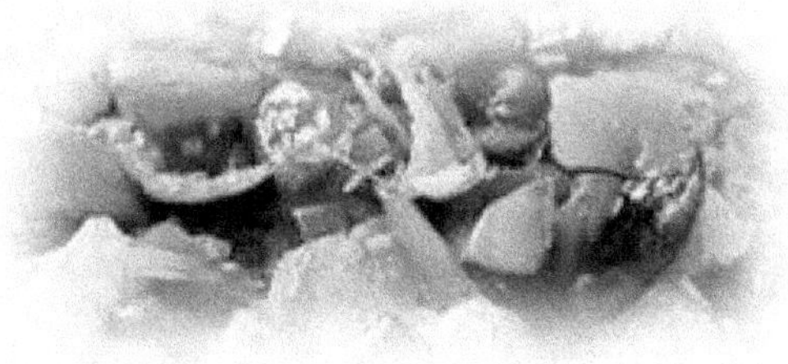

Disclaimer: The recipes contained in this cookbook are intended for personal use and enjoyment. The author and publisher are not responsible for any health issues or allergic reactions that may arise from the use of the ingredients or recipes provided. It is recommended that individuals with specific dietary concerns or restrictions consult a qualified healthcare professional.

DR. GRACE HESTER

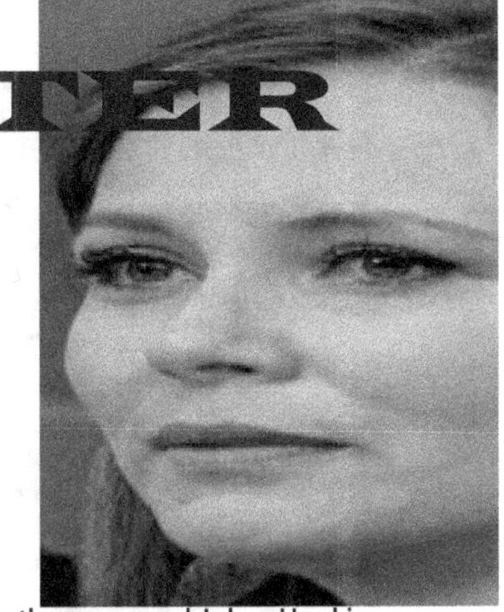

Dr. Grace Hester stands at the intersection of health, passion, and culinary excellence. A distinguished medical professional and accomplished nutritionist, she seamlessly weaves together her expertise to create a holistic approach to well-being.

Dr. Hester earned her medical degree from the renowned Johns Hopkins School of Medicine, consistently ranked among the top medical schools globally. Her commitment to advancing healthcare led her to prestigious positions at the Mayo Clinic, where she honed her skills in internal medicine. Driven by a desire to explore the profound connection between nutrition and overall health, she furthered her education at the Culinary Institute of America.

– With a deep understanding of both medicine and nutrition, Dr. Hester embarked on a mission to inspire others to embrace a healthier lifestyle. Her culinary journey– led to the creation of a series of cookbooks that blend the art of cooking with the science of nutrition. Each recipe is a testament to her commitment to flavor, nourishment, and well-being.

Currently, Dr. Hester serves as the Chief Nutritionist at the renowned Cleveland Clinic, where she continues to innovate in the field of nutritional medicine. Her groundbreaking work has been recognized not only within the medical community but also by a broader audience seeking practical and delicious ways to enhance their health.

B

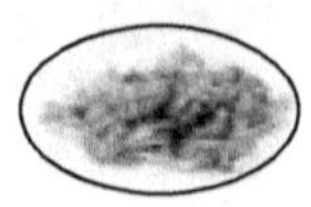 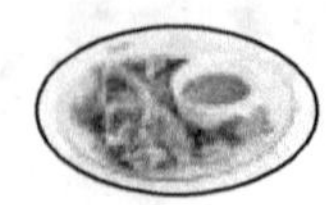 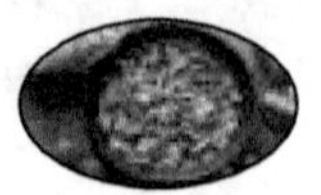

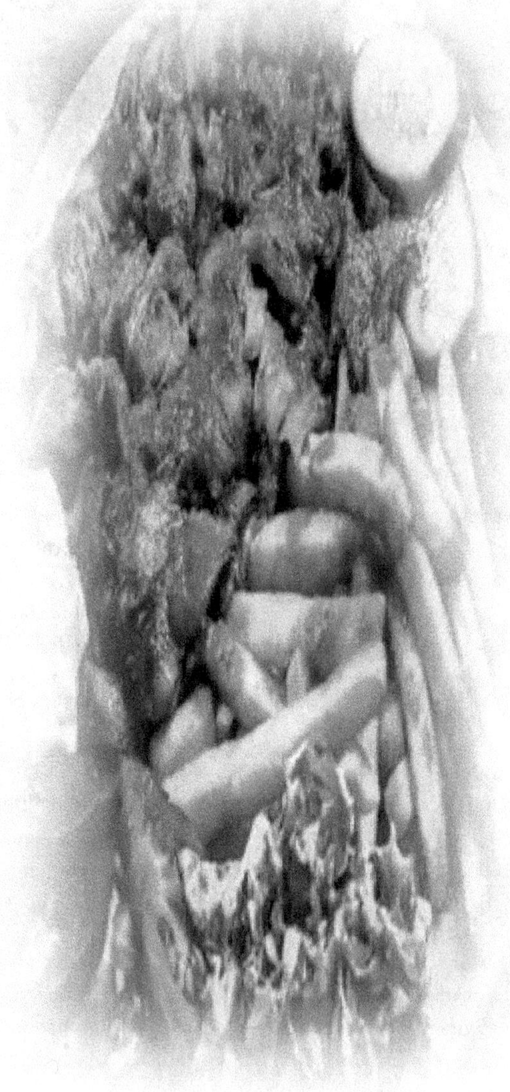

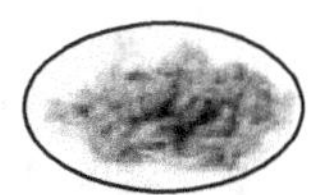 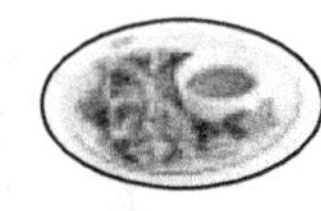 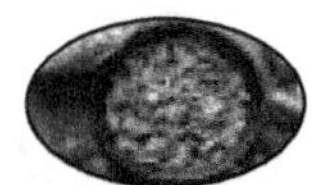

TABLE OF CONTENT

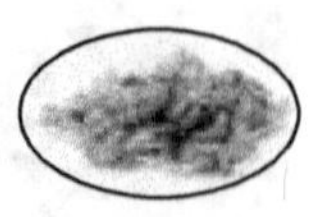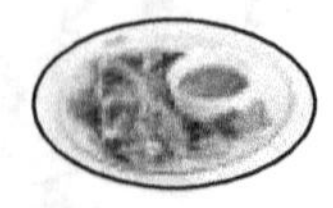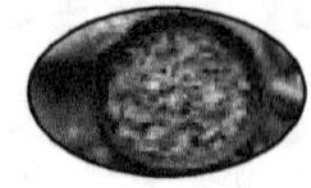

GESTATIONAL RECIPES FOR DINNER -------------------------------49

SNACKS AND LITTLE MEALS -------------------------------------67

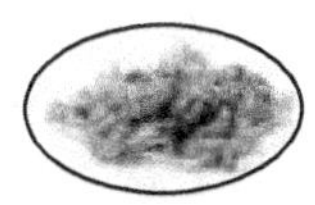
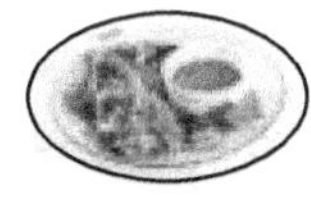
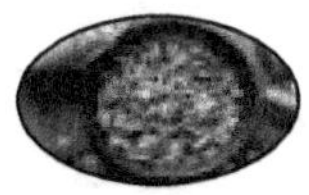

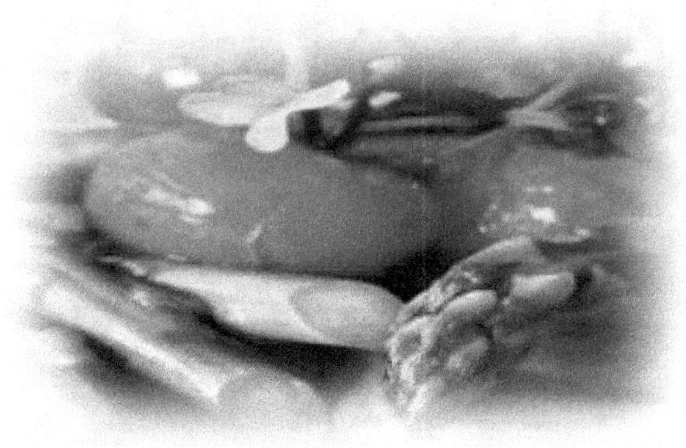

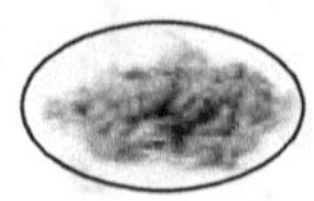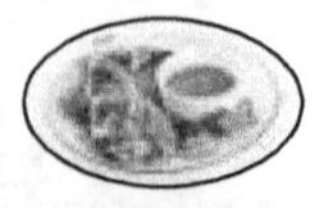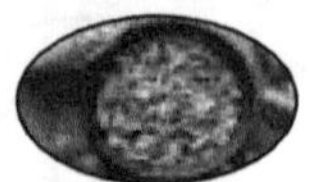

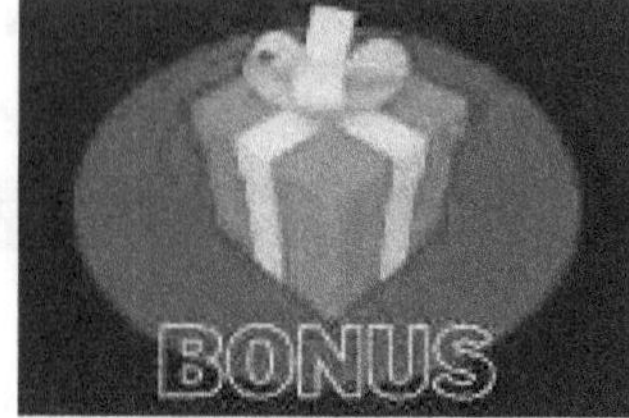

SCAN THE QR CODE TO GET YOUR FREE HOME MADE GREEN SMOOTHIE RECIPE BOOK

Your 20 days meal planner is attached at the end of the book. Enjoy!

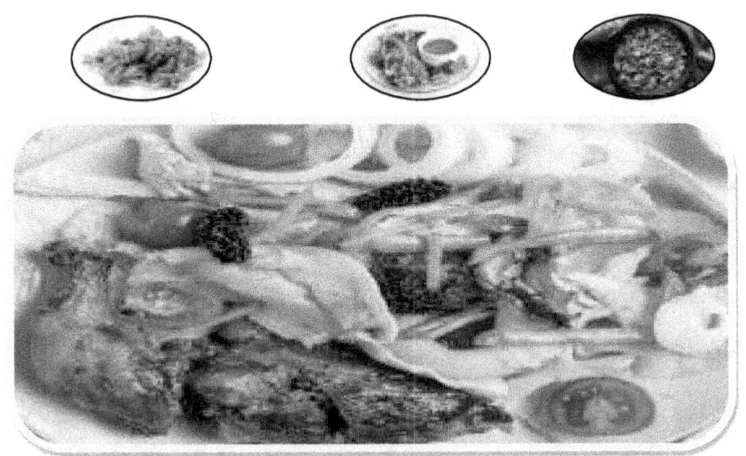

INTRODUCTION

There once was a woman named Sarah who lived in a world similar to our own. As she anticipated the birth of her first child, Sarah's life was characterized by happiness, love, and anticipation. Her days were spent daydreaming about the baby's name, nursery decor, and the precious moments she would soon enjoy with her child.

In the midst of the excitement, Sarah learned something unexpected that put her dreams in jeopardy. Her doctor said two words during a regular pregnancy visit that sent chills down her spine: "Gestational diabetes." When Sarah discovered that her path to motherhood had taken an unexpected turn, her heart sunk.–

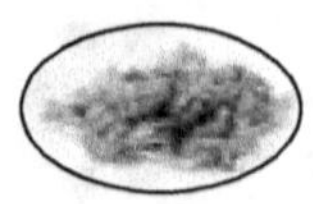 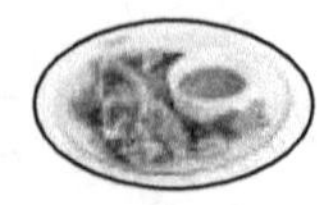 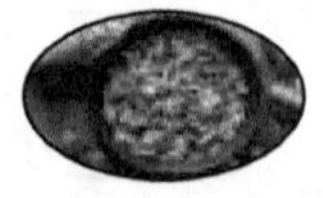

Pregnancy diabetes? What did that imply for her and the child she was carrying? Sarah learnt that this disease could result in issues during pregnancy and delivery, endangering the health of both her and her unborn child. She felt helpless and paralyzed with worry, fear, and helplessness.

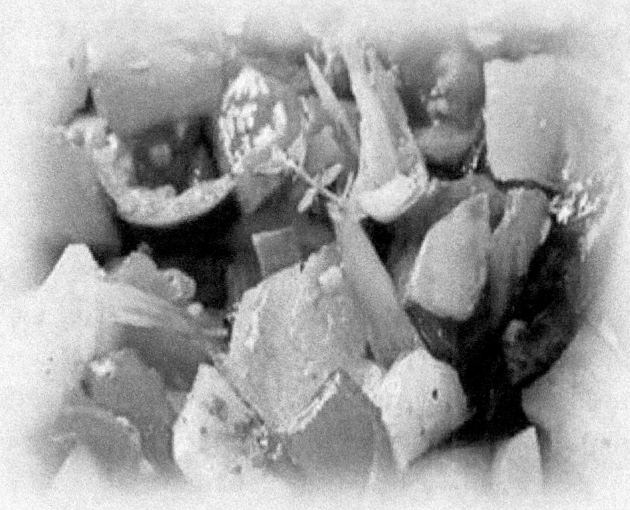

Sarah started her trek through the maze of medical advice, food restrictions, and lifestyle adjustments in search of answers. The internet was a sea of information, full of competing suggestions, difficult medical terminology, and tales of adversity. Sarah needed a lifeline and a light to aid her through this difficult terrain and protect the welfare of her child.

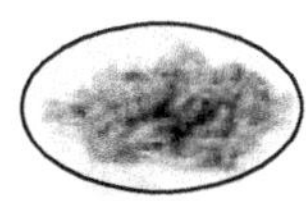 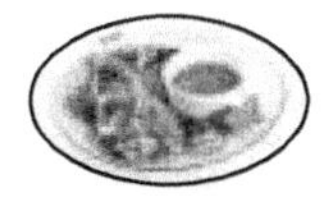 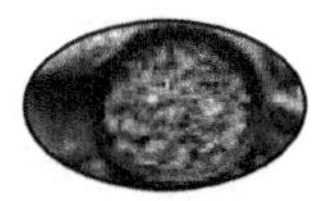

That's when she came across the "Gestational Diabetes Cookbook for Newly Diagnosed"—a wealth of information and encouragement written by specialists who had been in her position. Its name alone aroused her interest and provided a ray of hope. Uncertain of what she would discover, Sarah opened its pages with nervous hands.

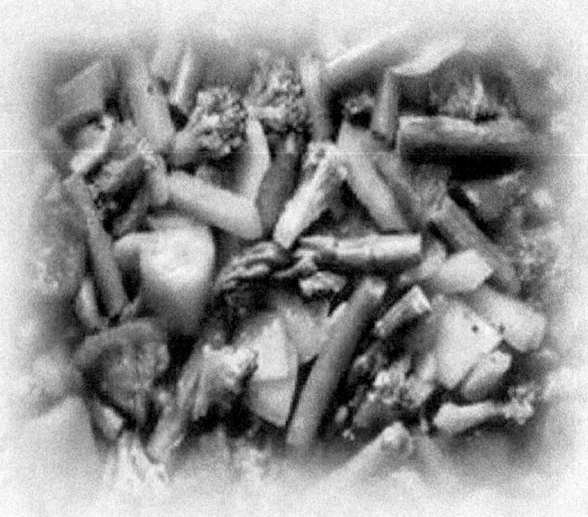

Sarah dug deeper into the cookbook and found a world of gastronomic pleasures catered to her particular requirements. The recipes were created to tantalize the taste buds while controlling blood sugar levels, not only to produce bland, unappealing meals. The cookbook promised variety and flavor without sacrificing her health or the health of her unborn child, with tantalizing breakfast selections, magnificent dinners, and guilt-free treats.–

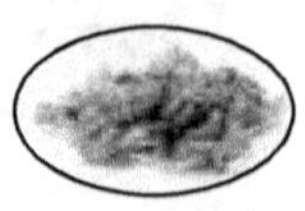 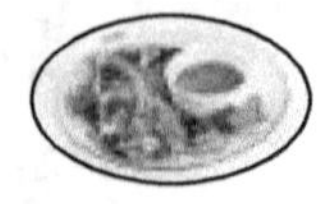 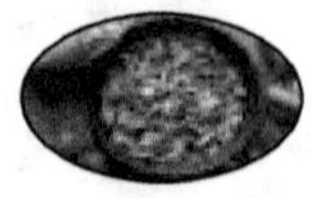

As Sarah started applying the cookbook's suggestions to her regular activities, its significance became clear. Each recipe included comprehensive nutritional information, suggestions for serving quantities, and management advice for her gestational diabetes. Sarah felt strong and in control as she was no longer trapped in the maze of dietary limitations.

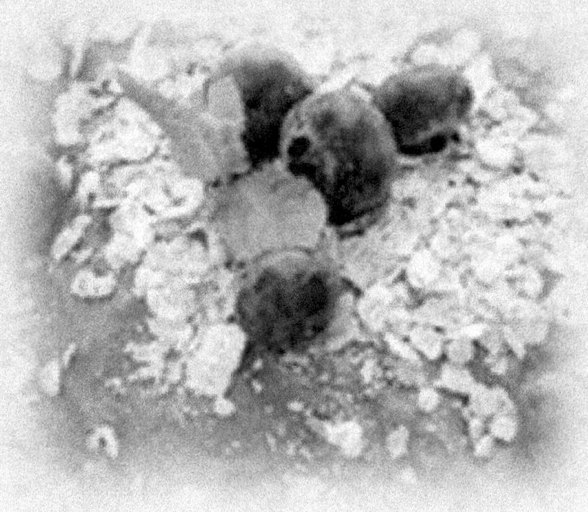

Sarah had a dramatic shift as the days and weeks passed. Her energy levels increased, and she had fewer desires for sweet foods. She felt better and more assured that she could control her situation. The fact that her monthly examinations revealed stable blood sugar levels and a developing, healthy baby was the most significant indication of improvement.–

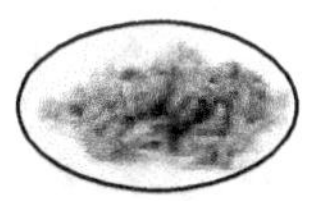 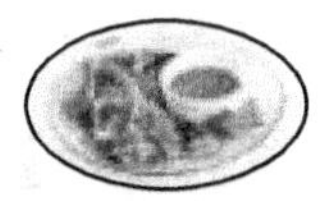 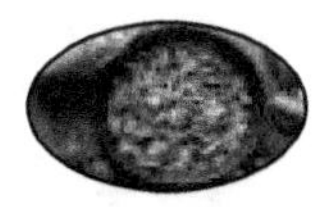

Sarah's tale was not an unusual occurrence. She discovered that she was able to relate to other mothers who had experienced comparable difficulties as she continued to follow the cookbook's instructions. They provided emotional support, recipe exchanges, and experience sharing. A single cookbook that had altered their lives brought together a community of resiliency, optimism, and tenacity.

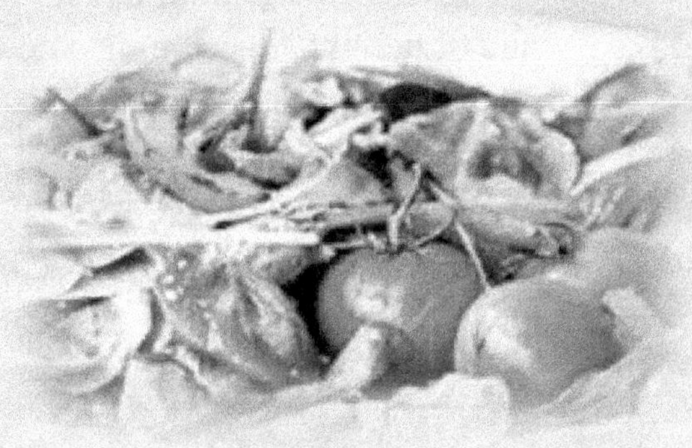

Beyond its mouthwatering meals, the "Gestational Diabetes Cookbook for Newly Diagnosed" had several advantages. Numerous women, including Sarah, found it to be a lifeline, providing them with a path to greater health and promising futures for their offspring. It wasn't only about controlling gestational diabetes; it was also about reversing its effects and making sure their unborn children got off to a safe, healthy start.–

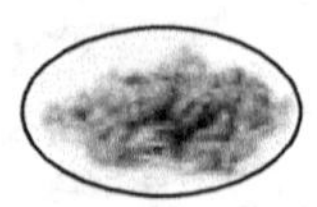 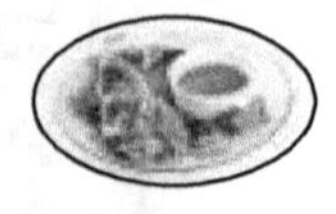 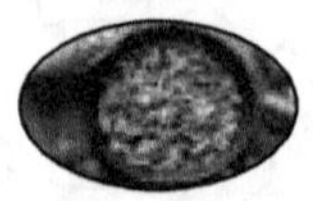

Sarah's doctor was impressed with her development as the due date drew near. What had once been an unclear diagnosis has changed into a journey of empowerment and hope. Sarah's experience was proof of the value of the cookbook, showing that gestational diabetes could be controlled and even reversed with the correct information and assistance.

Finally, Sarah got to hold her lovely child in her arms. In addition to being tears of delight at becoming a new mother, they were also tears of triumph against adversity. Thanks to the "Gestational Diabetes Cookbook for Newly Diagnosed," Sarah not only gave birth to a healthy child but also developed a fresh understanding of the value of education, community, and delectable, diabetes-friendly food.

So, my reader, the inspirational prologue to the priceless book "Gestational Diabetes Cookbook for Newly Diagnosed" that is Sarah's tale and her transformational experience with gestational diabetes. You'll discover not only a selection of delicious recipes but also the assurance of hope, good health, and a better future for moms and their priceless children within its pages. Join us as we explore this incredible cookbook's culinary delights and game-changing advantages, learning how it can make your battle with gestational diabetes into a story of joy and victory.

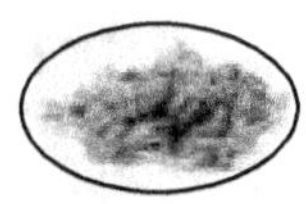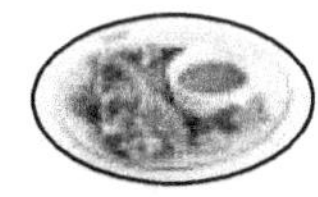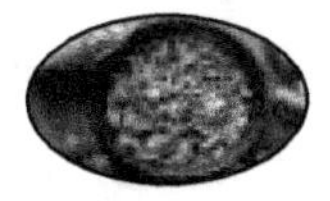

BEING CONSCIOUS OF GESTATIONAL DIABETES

Pregnant women who have gestational diabetes mellitus (GDM) experience elevated blood sugar levels throughout pregnancy. Both the mother and the child may suffer grave health consequences as a result of this disorder. For the health of both mother and child, it is essential to comprehend the origins, risk factors, and significance of controlling gestational diabetes.

Risk elements

A woman is more likely to have gestational diabetes if certain conditions exist. These risk elements consist of:

Age: Women over the age of 25, especially those over 35, are more at risk.

Family history: The risk of acquiring GDM is higher if diabetes runs in the family.

Obesity: Before becoming pregnant, being overweight or obese increases the risk.–

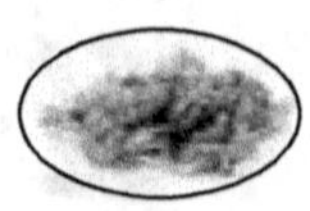 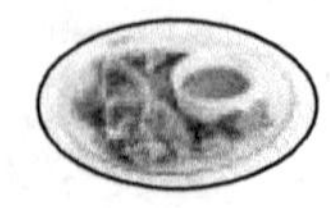 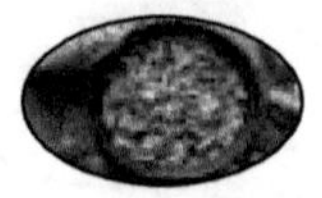

Previous GDM: Women who have experienced gestational diabetes during pregnancy are more likely to experience it once more.

PCOS: Women who have PCOS are at increased risk of developing GDM.

Glycemic History: Prior pregnancy with prediabetes or a history of high blood sugar levels increases the risk.

Multiple Pregnancies: Having twins or more increases your risk of developing GDM.

Causes:

Although the precise causes of gestational diabetes are not entirely understood, it is believed that a number of hormonal, genetic, and lifestyle variables are involved. The hormones in the body fluctuate significantly during pregnancy, and some of these hormones may interact with insulin, which controls blood sugar levels.

The mother's body's ability to utilize insulin can be hampered by hormones produced by the placenta, which supplies nourishment to the growing fetus. In order to make up for this, the mother's pancreas must generate extra insulin. Gestational diabetes develops if the pancreas is unable to handle this additional demand, which causes blood sugar levels to rise.–

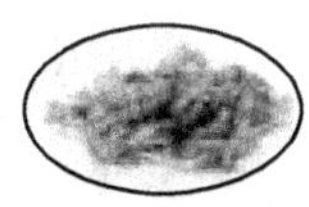 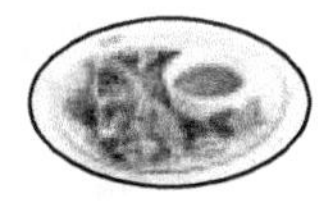 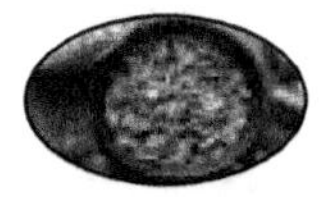

The significance of controlling gestational diabetes

Health of the Mother: If gestational diabetes is not managed, it can cause complications for the mother's health, such as high blood pressure, preeclampsia (a serious illness that can be fatal), and a higher risk of acquiring type 2 diabetes in the future.

Health of the Baby: Several issues, such as: High blood sugar levels in the mother can be transmitted to the baby through the placenta.

Macrosomia: Babies born to moms with GDM are frequently bigger than typical, which raises the possibility of harm during delivery.

Hypoglycemia: The newborn's blood sugar levels may dangerously fall after birth.

Respiratory Distress Syndrome: GDM can increase the likelihood that a baby will experience breathing issues.–

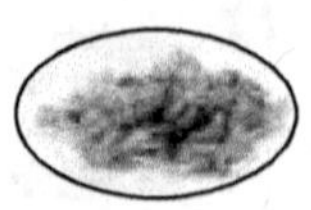 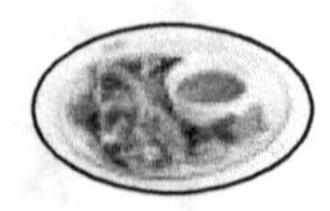 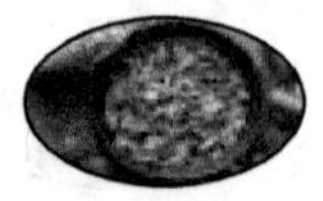

Jaundice can result from high bilirubin levels in a baby's blood.

Type 2 Diabetes: Children born to moms who have GDM are more likely to develop type 2 diabetes in the future.

Complications during birth: Keeping blood sugar levels under control during pregnancy lowers the likelihood of problems during delivery, such as the necessity for a cesarean section.

Long-Term Health: Proper gestational diabetes management lowers the likelihood that both the mother and the fetus may go on to develop type 2 diabetes in the future.

Gestational diabetes management:

For a good pregnancy and healthy infant, gestational diabetes must be effectively managed. Here are some essential methods for controlling GDM:

Monitoring Blood Sugar Levels: Maintaining blood sugar levels within a healthy range requires regular monitoring of these levels. Checking your blood sugar regularly is usually necessary, especially after meals.–

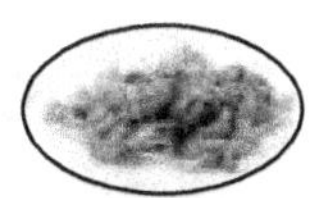 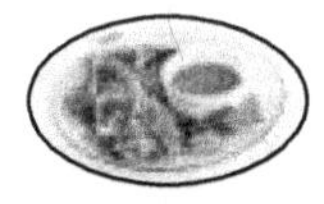 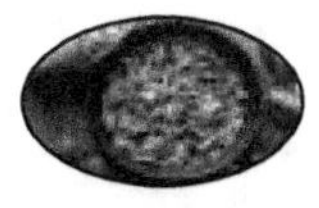

Healthy Eating: Complex carbohydrates, fiber, lean proteins, and healthy fats should all be included in a balanced diet to help control blood sugar levels. A licensed dietician can offer suggestions for meal preparation.

Exercise routinely: Maintaining an active lifestyle can aid with blood sugar management. However, it's crucial to speak with a healthcare professional to choose a safe and suitable fitness program during pregnancy.

Insulin or medication: In some circumstances, controlling blood sugar levels by diet and exercise alone may not be enough. A healthcare professional may recommend insulin injections or oral medicine.

Prenatal visits that are routine: Regular prenatal checkups enable medical professionals to keep a close eye on both the mother's and the unborn child's health.

Counseling and support: Attending support meetings or getting therapy might help you deal with the emotional effects of gestational diabetes.–

Planning for birth: Because gestational diabetes can have an impact on the timing and mode of birth, it's imperative to talk with a healthcare professional about delivery alternatives.–

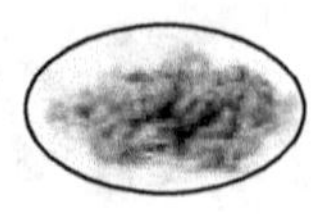 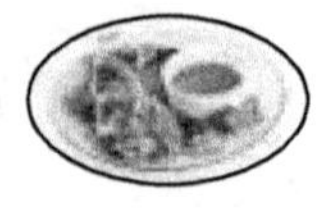 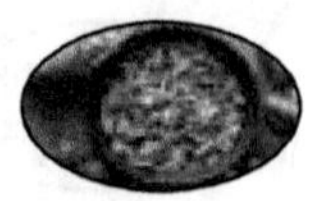

Planning meals and monitoring portions

Portion control and meal preparation for gestational diabetes

A kind of diabetes known as gestational diabetes mellitus (GDM) appears during pregnancy. Planning meals and controlling portions properly are crucial parts of treating gestational diabetes to protect the mother's and the unborn child's health. The tactics for building a balanced plate, comprehending carbs, controlling portion sizes, and timing meals are covered in this article.

How to Balance a Plate:

The secret to controlling blood sugar levels is a balanced meal. Try to include a range of items from several food categories on your plate:–

Vegetables: Non-starchy vegetables like leafy greens, broccoli, and cauliflower should make about half of your meal. These have a high fiber content and few carbohydrates, which helps control blood sugar.

—

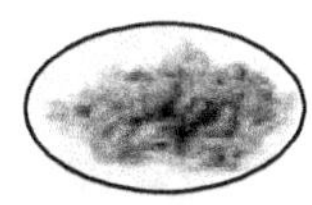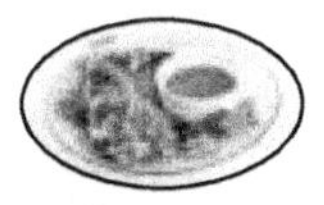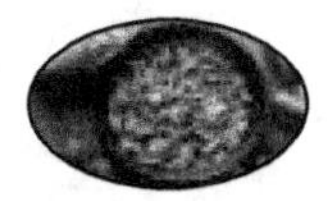

Lean proteins like chicken, fish, tofu, or beans should make up a quarter of your dish. Both vital nutrients and blood sugar stabilization are provided by protein.

Carbohydrates: Put carbohydrates on the last part of your plate. Pick complex carbs like legumes and whole grains like brown rice, quinoa, and whole wheat pasta. These take longer than simple carbohydrates to release sugar into your system.

Fats: Include in moderation healthy fats like avocado, olive oil, and almonds. They may contribute to feeling full and enjoying your meal more generally.

Recognizing Carbohydrates

Blood sugar levels are most significantly influenced by carbohydrates. You must keep an eye on and manage your carbohydrate intake:

Count Carbs: Consult a certified dietician to ascertain how many carbohydrates you require each day. They will work with you to develop a carbohydrate counting strategy that meets your needs.–

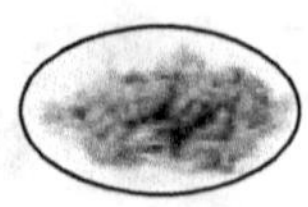 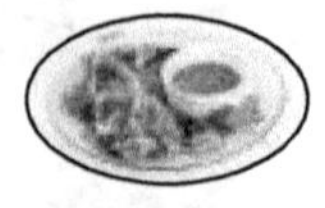 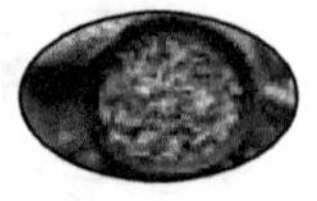

Pick Wisely: Rather than simple sugars, choose complex carbs. Avoid processed foods, fizzy drinks, and sweets. Place a priority on whole, unprocessed foods.

Whole grains, veggies, and legumes are examples of foods high in fiber that can help control blood sugar levels. Per day, aim for at least 25 grams of fiber.

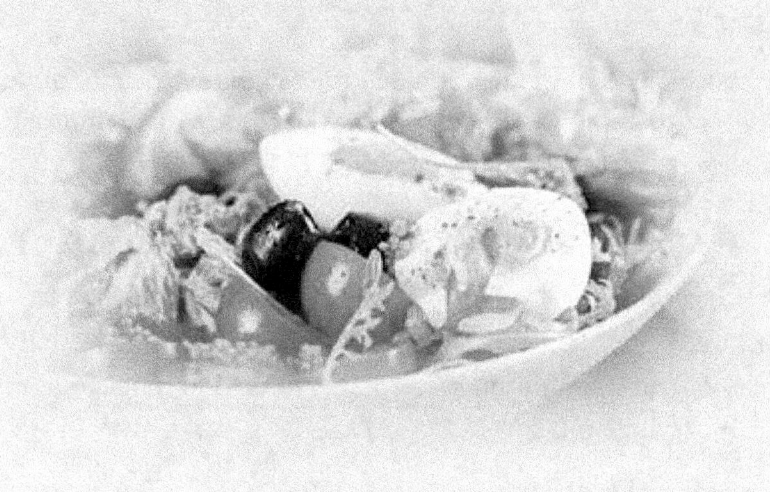

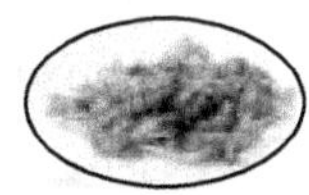 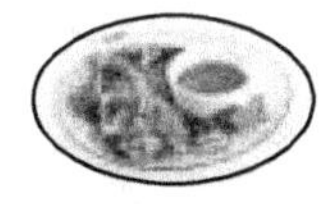 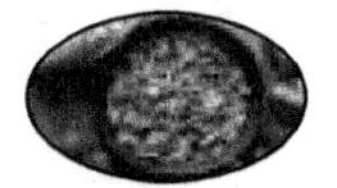

Serving Sizes:

Controlling one's intake is essential for managing gestational diabetes:

Use Measuring Tools: To correctly portion your meals, buy measuring cups and a food scale. This guarantees that you aren't consuming more carbohydrates than is healthy.

Small, Regular Meals: Throughout the day, eating small, wholesome meals might help reduce blood sugar increases. To keep your levels consistent, try to eat every two to three hours.

How to Time Your Meals:

Blood sugar levels can be impacted by when you eat:

Maintain a consistent mealtime routine by following it. Your body can better control blood sugar levels if you eat at the same times every day.–

Check Blood Sugar Levels After Meals: Check your blood sugar levels after meals to see how various foods influence you. This might assist you in modifying your diet as necessary.–

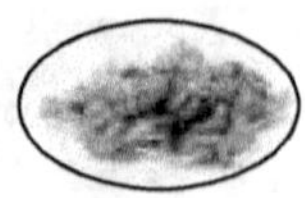 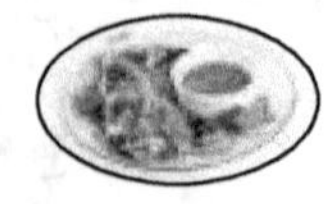 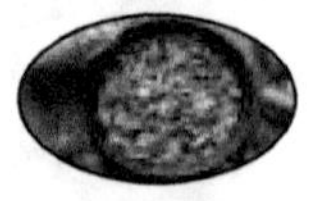

A quick, protein-rich snack before bed can help control blood sugar levels the following morning.

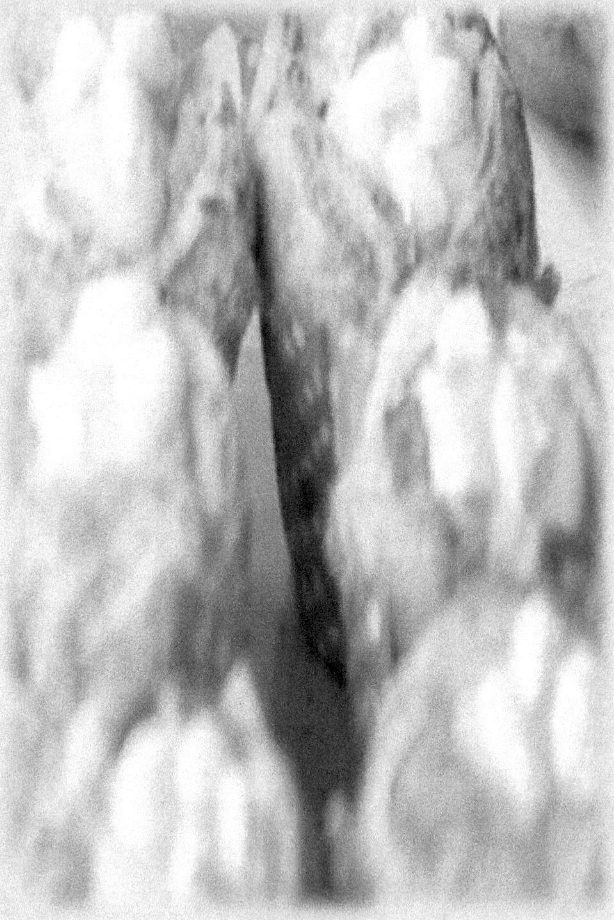

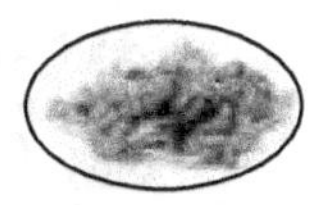 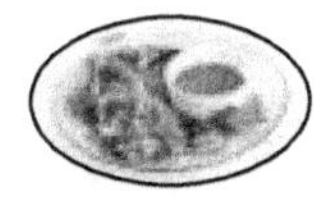 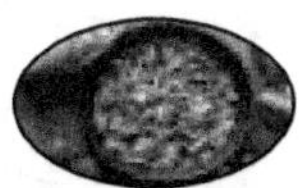

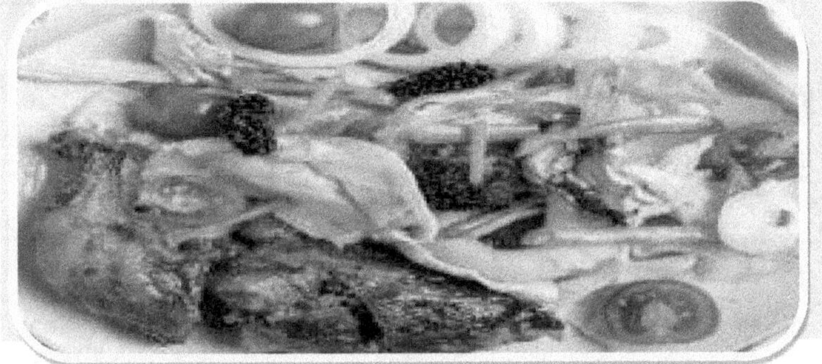

Gestational Recipes for breakfast

Greek yogurt parfait

INGREDIENTS:

- 1/2 cup plain Greek yogurt
- 14 cup of fresh berries
- 1 tablespoon of chopped nuts, such as walnuts or almonds
- One teaspoon of optional honey
- In a glass, arrange yogurt, berries, and nuts.
- If desired, drizzle with honey.—

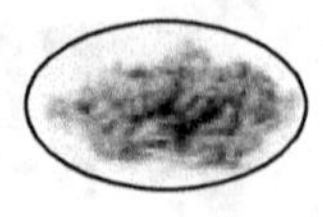 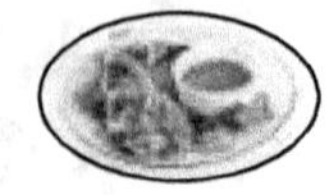 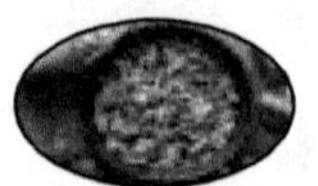

Approximate nutritional value:

200 calories

20g carbs

12g of protein

Preparation Time: 5 minutes

Vegetable Omelet

INGREDIENTS:

- two eggs, big
- 14 cup of bell peppers, diced
- tomato dice, one-fourth cup
- 2 tablespoons of onions, diced
- pepper and salt as desired

PREPARATION:

Eggs are whisked before being added to a hot nonstick skillet.

Season with salt and pepper, then add the vegetables and cook until done.–

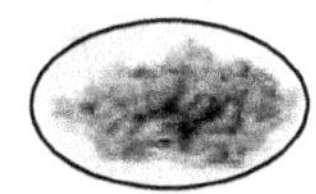 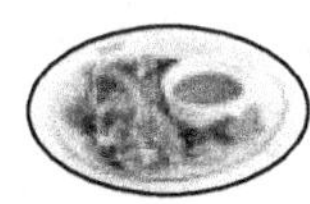 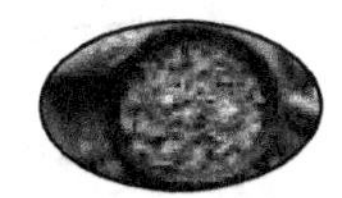

- 220 calories
- 7g carbs
- 14g of protein
- 10 minutes for cooking

Chia pudding made the night before:

INGREDIENTS:

- Chia seeds, 2 tablespoons
- 1 cup of almond milk without sugar
- a smidge of vanilla extract
- a half-cup of cut strawberries

PREPARATION:

In a container, combine vanilla, almond milk, and chia seeds.

Overnight refrigerate.

Prior to serving, garnish with strawberries.

Approximate nutritional value:

180 calories

17g carbs

6g protein

5 minutes of cooking plus overnight refrigeration

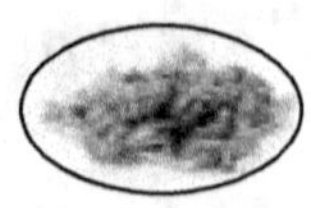 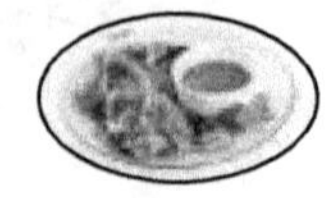 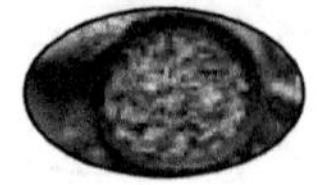

Toast with avocado:

INGREDIENTS:

- 1 piece of whole-wheat bread
- ripe avocado, half
- juice from a lemon squeeze
- pepper and salt as desired

Prepare the bread by toasting it.

Combine salt, pepper, and lemon juice in an avocado mash.

Apply to toast.

APPROXIMATE NUTRITIONAL VALUE:

- 200 calories; 18g carbs
- 4g. protein

Preparation Time: 5 minutes

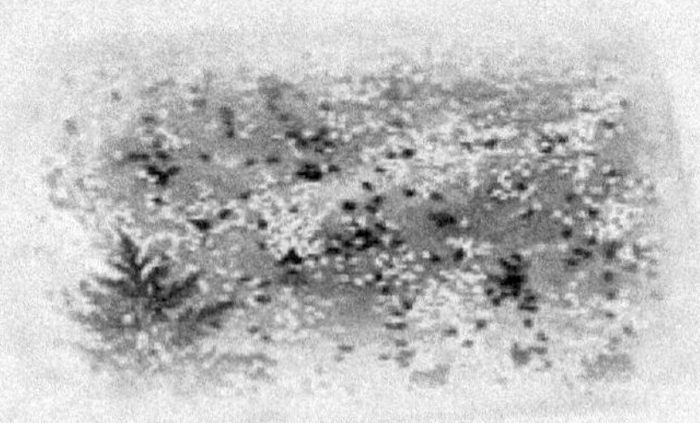

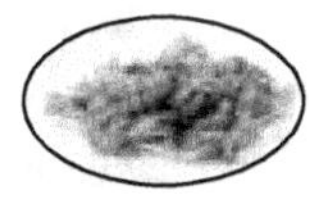 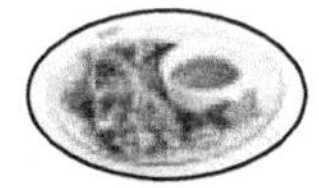 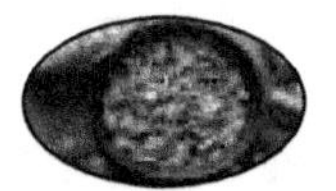

Berries and Cottage Cheese:

INGREDIENTS:

- Low-fat cottage cheese, half a cup
- 14 cup of berries in general
- One teaspoon of optional honey

PREPARATION:

Add berries to the cottage cheese.

If desired, drizzle with honey.

APPROXIMATE NUTRITIONAL VALUE:

180 calories; 18g carbs

15g of protein

Preparation Time: 5 minutes–

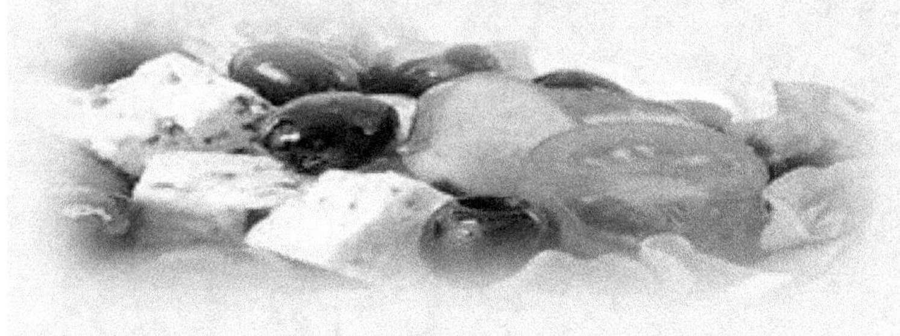

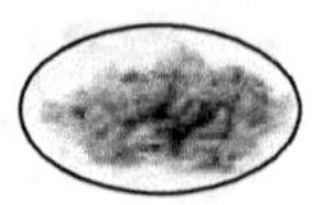 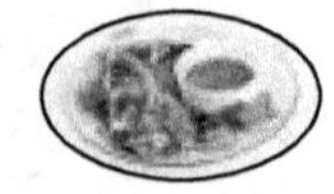 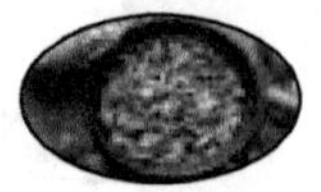

Breakfast bowl with quinoa:

INGREDIENTS:

- half a cup of cooked quinoa.
- 14 cup of banana slices
- 1 tablespoon of nuts, chopped
- 1 spoonful of unsweetened Greek yogurt
- 0.5 teaspoons of optional honey

PREPARATION:

In a bowl, arrange the quinoa, banana, almonds, and yogurt.

If desired, drizzle with honey.

APPROXIMATE NUTRITIONAL VALUE:

250 calories

35g of carbs

8g protein

Cooking time, including quinoa cooking, is 15 minutes.–

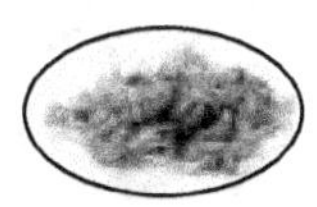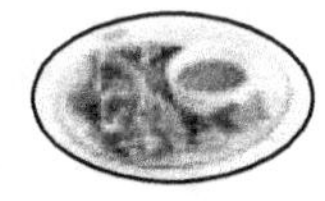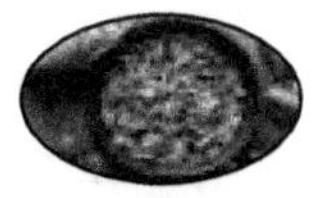

Smoothie with peanut butter and bananas:

INGREDIENTS:

- One little, ripe banana
- 2 tablespoons of unsweetened peanut butter
- 12 cup almond milk without sugar
- Ice cubes, if desired

PREPARATION:

All ingredients should be smoothly combined.

Approximate nutritional value:

280 calories; 26g carbs

8g protein

Preparation Time: 5 minutes

—

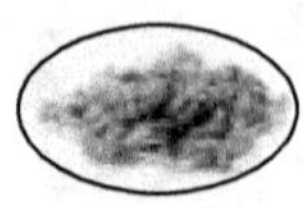 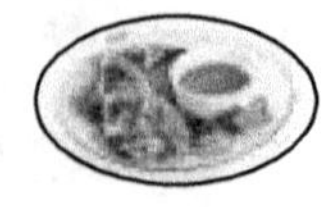 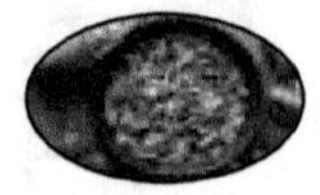

Egg Muffins with Spinach and Feta:

INGREDIENTS:

- 4 eggs, big
- Chopped spinach, half a cup
- 1/4 cup feta cheese crumbles
- pepper and salt as desired

PREPARATION:

Salt, pepper, feta, spinach, and eggs are whisked together.

Bake for 15-20 minutes at 350°F (175°C) in muffin tins.

Approximate nutritional value:

120 calories per muffin

1g of carbs

9g protein

20 minutes for cooking–

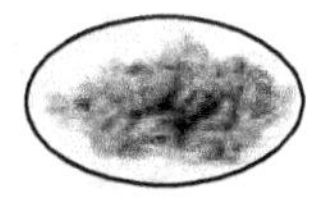 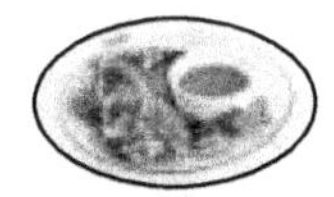 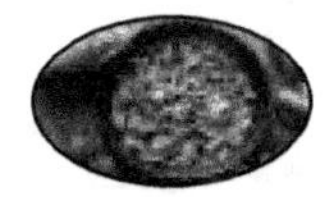

Blended Berry and Almond Bowl

INGREDIENTS:

- half a cup of mixed frozen berries.
- 1/4 cup of almond milk without sugar
- Almond butter, two tablespoons

Fresh berries, chia seeds, and sliced almonds are the toppings.

Berry, almond milk, and almond butter should be blended till smooth before serving.

Pour into a bowl, then top with garnishes.

APPROXIMATE NUTRITIONAL VALUE:

300 calories

23g carbs

9g protein

Preparation Time: 5 minutes

—

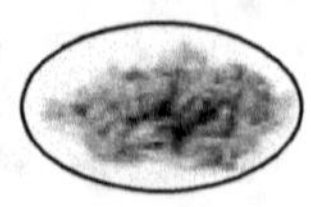 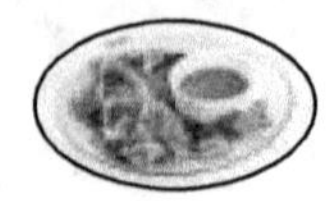 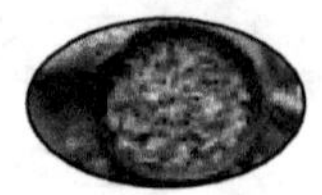

Wholesome pancakes

INGREDIENTS:

- 1/2 cup pancake mix made with healthy grains
- 14 cup of plain applesauce
- 1/4 cup of almond milk without sugar
- half a teaspoon of cinnamon

Mix the pancake mix, applesauce, almond milk, and cinnamon in a bowl.

Cook till golden brown using a nonstick skillet.

APPROXIMATE NUTRITIONAL VALUE:

250 calories (for two pancakes)

50g carbs

6g protein

10 minutes for cooking

To adapt these recipes to your unique nutritional requirements, keep an eye on portion amounts and speak with a healthcare provider.–

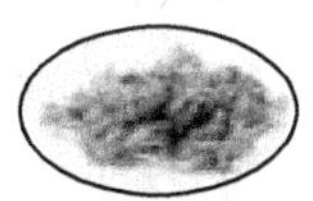 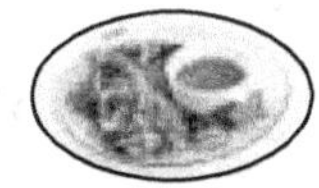 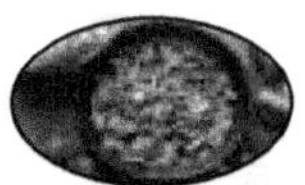

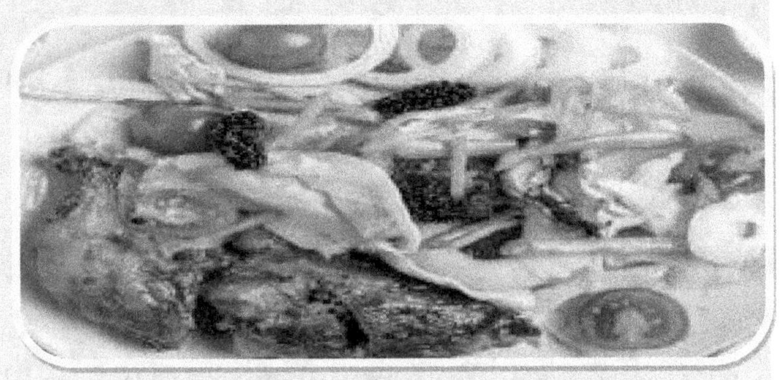

Gestational meals recipes

Grilled chicken salad

INGREDIENTS:

- 4 ounces of skinless, boneless chicken breast
- two cups of greens for a mixed salad
- Half a cup of cherry tomatoes
- sliced 1/4 cup of cucumber
- 2/TBS of olive oil
- Balsamic vinegar, 1 tablespoon
- pepper and salt as desired

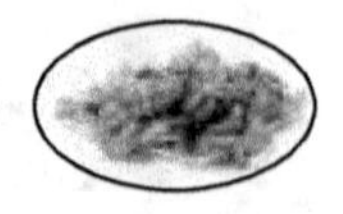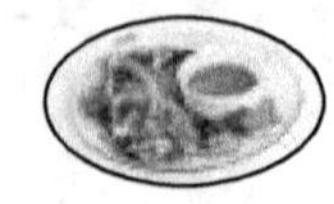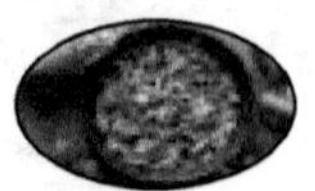

Salt and pepper the chicken, then grill it for 6 to 8 minutes on each side, or until it is thoroughly cooked.

Cut up the grilled chicken.

Salad greens, cherry tomatoes, and cucumber should all be combined in a bowl.

Add balsamic vinegar and olive oil before adding the grilled chicken.

VALUE NUTRITIVE (PER SERVING):

320 calories

30g of protein

8g of carbohydrates

2g of fiber

20 minutes for cooking–

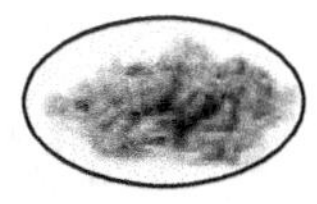 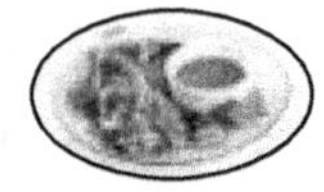 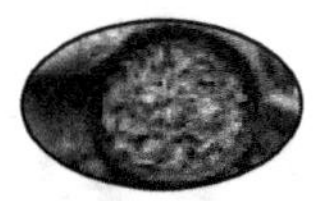

Bowl of quinoa and black beans

INGREDIENTS:

- 0.5 cups of quinoa
- one water cup
- 1/2 cup canned, rinsed black beans
- 1/4 cup of kernels of corn
- chopped 1/4 cup red bell pepper
- 1 cup salsa
- 1 tablespoon chopped fresh cilantro

PREPARATION:

Quinoa should be rinsed before being mixed with water in a pan. Turn heat down, cover, and simmer for 15 minutes after bringing to a boil.

With a fork, fluff cooked quinoa and allow it to cool.

Quinoa, black beans, corn, red bell pepper, and salsa should be combined in a bowl.

Add fresh cilantro on top.–

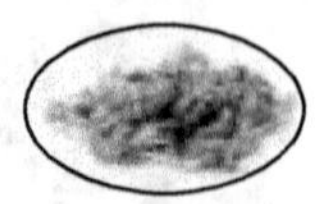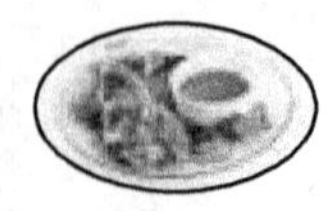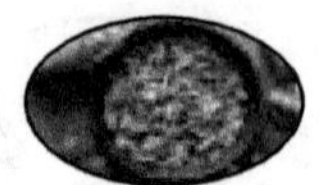

- 330 calories
- 12g of protein
- 59g of carbohydrates
- 10g of fiber
- 20 minutes for cooking

Fish with asparagus

INGREDIENTS:

- Salmon fillet, 4 oz.
- a half-bunch of asparagus
- 1 tablespoon of olive oil
- Sliced lemon, half
- pepper and salt as desired

PREPARATION:

Set the oven's temperature to 400°F (200°C).

Salmon and asparagus should be put on a baking pan.

Olive oil should be drizzled over the dish before adding salt and pepper and lemon slices.

Cook salmon for 15 to 20 minutes, or until it flakes easily.–

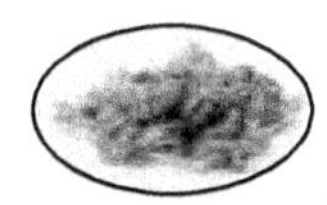 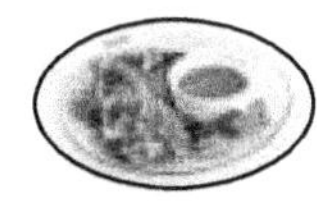 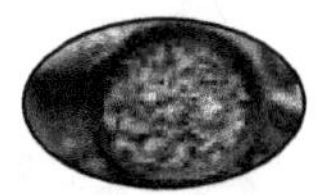

- 290 calories
- 24g of protein
- 5g of carbohydrates
- 2g of fiber

20 minutes for cooking

Wrap with turkey and avocado

INGREDIENTS:

- 4 ounce slices of turkey breast
- one whole-wheat tortilla
- 1/4 sliced avocado
- 4 cups of spinach leaves
- 1-tablespoon Greek yogurt
- Dijon mustard, 1/2 teaspoon

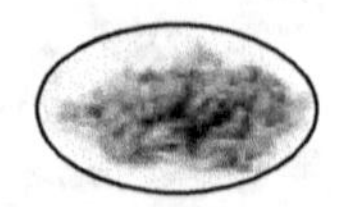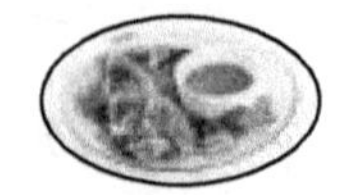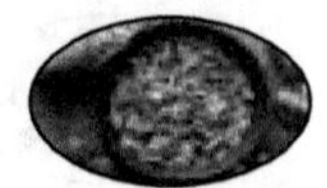

Spread the Greek yogurt and Dijon mustard evenly over the tortilla.

Slices of turkey, avocado, and spinach are layered.

Cut the tortilla in half after securely rolling it up.

Value nutritive (per serving):

- 320 calories
- 25g of protein
- 25g of carbohydrates
- 7g of fiber

10 minutes for cooking

Vegetable and Lentil Soup

INGREDIENTS:

- Dry green or brown lentils, 1/2 cup
- 2 cups of low-sodium vegetable broth 1 cup of chopped carrots
- chopped celery in a half cup–

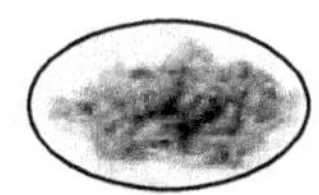 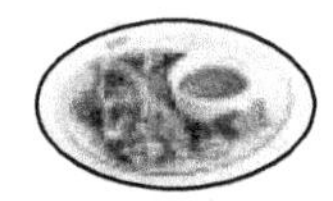 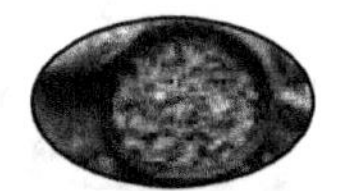

- 1/2 cup diced onion
- Olive oil, 1/2 tsp.
- 12 teaspoon cumin
- pepper and salt as desired

PREPARATION:

Lentils should be rinsed and stored.

Olive oil should be used to sauté celery, onions, and carrots in a big saucepan until they are soft.

Add cumin, salt, pepper, lentils, and vegetable broth. Boil for a few minutes, then turn down the heat and simmer for 20 to 25 minutes.

Value nutritive (per serving):

250 calories

15g of protein

45g of carbohydrates

12g of fiber

30 minutes for cooking–

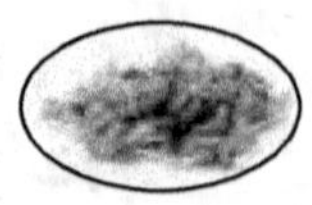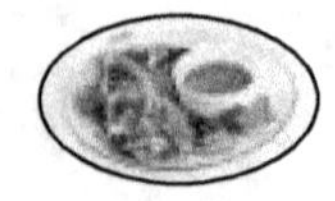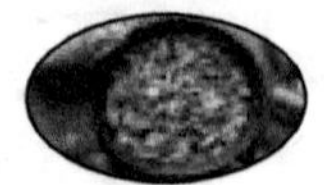

Stir-Fried Tofu

INGREDIENTS:

Cubed 4 ounces of firm tofu, 1 cup of broccoli florets

Snap peas and chopped half a cup of bell peppers

Low-sodium soy sauce, 1 tablespoon

minced 1/2 teaspoon each of ginger, garlic, and sesame oil.

PREPARATION:

Tofu cubes are added to a skillet of heated sesame oil. Brown food in the oven.

Stir in the ginger, garlic, and soy sauce before adding the vegetables.

Vegetables should be cooked for 5-7 minutes or until soft.

Value nutritive (per serving):

- 280 calories
- 16g of protein
- 16g of carbohydrates
- 5g of fiber

15 minutes for cooking–

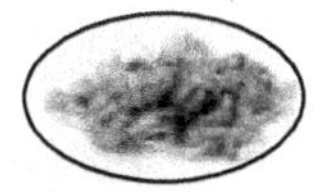 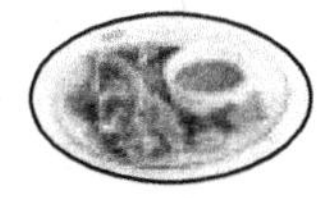 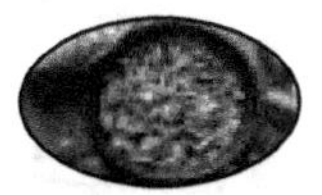

Salad of Greek Quinoa

0.5 cups of quinoa

one water cup

diced 1/4 cup cucumber

2 tablespoons of finely chopped red onion, 2 tablespoons of crumbled feta cheese, 2 tablespoons of pitted and sliced Kalamata olives, and 1/4 cup cherry tomatoes

1 tablespoon of olive oil

1-tablespoon lemon juice

Oregano, dried, 12 tsp.

PREPARATION:

Quinoa should be rinsed before being mixed with water in a pan. Turn heat down, cover, and simmer for 15 minutes after bringing to a boil.

With a fork, fluff cooked quinoa and allow it to cool.

Quinoa, cucumber, cherry tomatoes, red onion, feta cheese, and olives should all be combined in a bowl.

Olive oil, lemon juice, and dried oregano should be added.

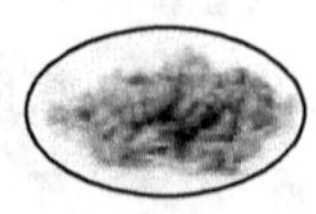 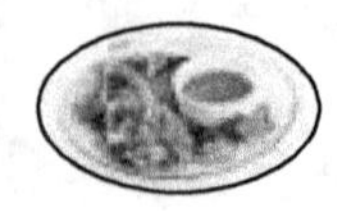 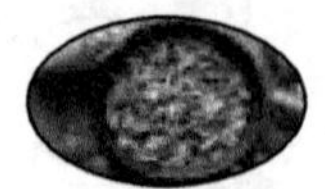

Value nutritive (per serving):

330 calories

9g protein

43g of carbohydrates

5g of fiber

20 minutes for cooking

Omelette with eggs and spinach

INGREDIENTS:

- two huge eggs
- one cup of new spinach
- diced 1/4 cup bell peppers
- sliced 1/4 cup of mushrooms
- 14 cup of low-fat cheese, shredded
- frying oil
- pepper and salt as desired–

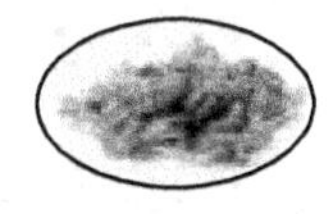 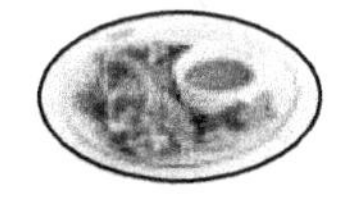 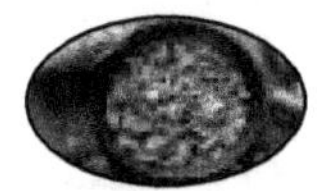

PREPARATION:

After thoroughly whisking your eggs, ensure you add to taste salt and pepper.

Cooking spray is added to a non-stick skillet and heated over medium heat.

Add the mushrooms and bell peppers, and cook them both until soft.

Add spinach, whisked eggs, and cheese before covering the vegetables.

Fold the omelette in half after cooking the eggs until they are set.

VALUE NUTRITIVE (PER SERVING):

280 calories

18g of protein

6g of carbohydrates

2g of fiber

10 minutes for cooking

—

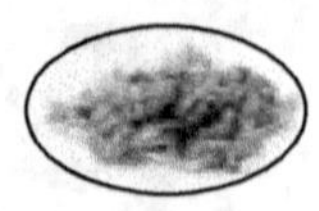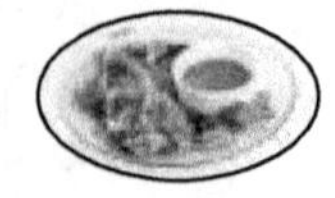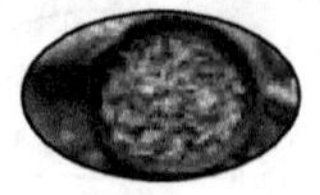

Stir-Fried Turkey and Veggies

INGREDIENTS:

- Lean ground turkey, 4 ounces
- broccoli florets in a cup
- Snap peas, half a cup
- sliced 1/2 cup of carrots
- Low-sodium soy sauce, 14 cup
- 1/8 teaspoon minced ginger
- minced 1/2 tsp of garlic, 1/2 tsp of sesame oil

PREPARATION:

Ground turkey is added to a pan with heated sesame oil. Brown food in the oven.

Stir in the ginger, garlic, and soy sauce before adding the vegetables.

Vegetables should be cooked for 5-7 minutes or until soft.

Value nutritive (per serving):

280 calories

26g of protein–

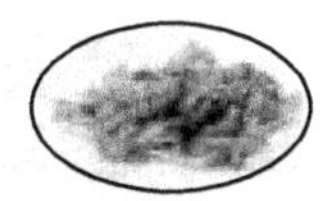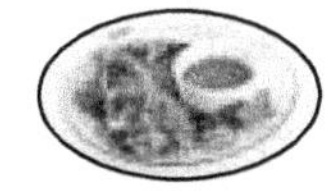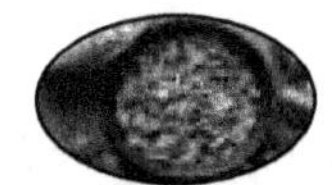

15g of carbohydrates

5g of fiber

15 minutes for cooking

Quiche with spinach and mushrooms

- a single whole-wheat pie crust
- 1 cup chopped fresh spinach
- Sliced mushrooms, 4 large eggs, and half a cup
- one cup of nonfat milk
- 14 cup of low-fat cheese, shredded
- pepper and salt as desired

Set the oven's temperature to 350°F (175°C).

Sauté spinach and mushrooms in a skillet until the spinach wilts.

Thoroughly stair the eggs, likewise the milk, salt, and pepper in a big bowl.

Put the cheese and the egg mixture on top of the sautéed vegetables in the pie shell.

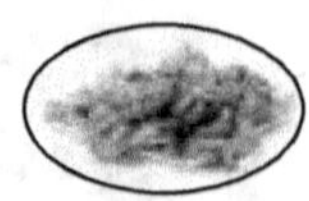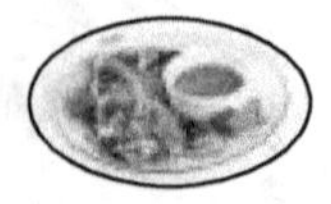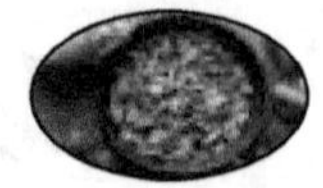

Bake until firm, about 35 to 40 minutes.

Value nutritive (per serving):

320 calories

15g of protein

25g of carbohydrates

3g of fiber

50 minutes for cooking

Ten lunch recipes for women with gestational diabetes are listed below. Enjoy your wholesome food!

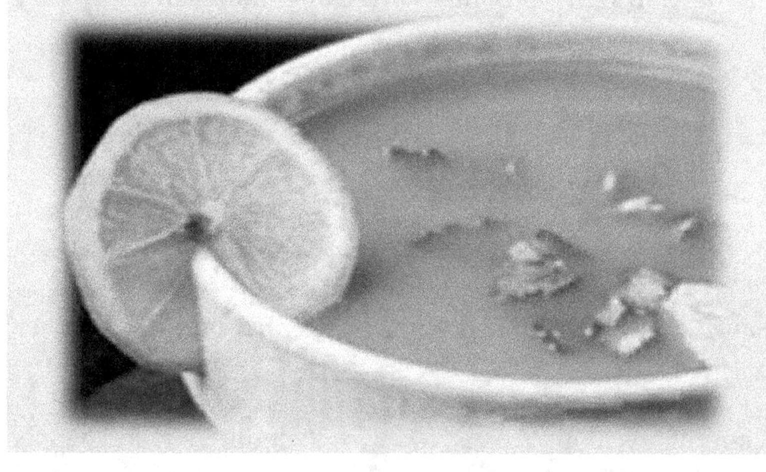

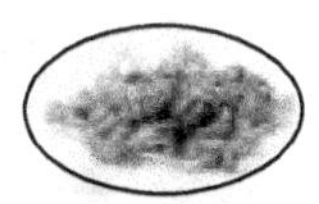 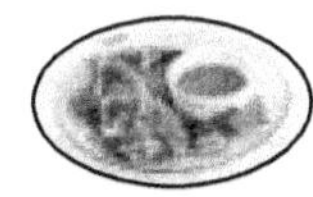 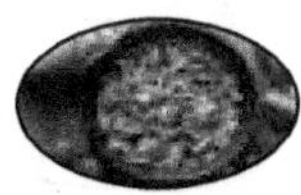

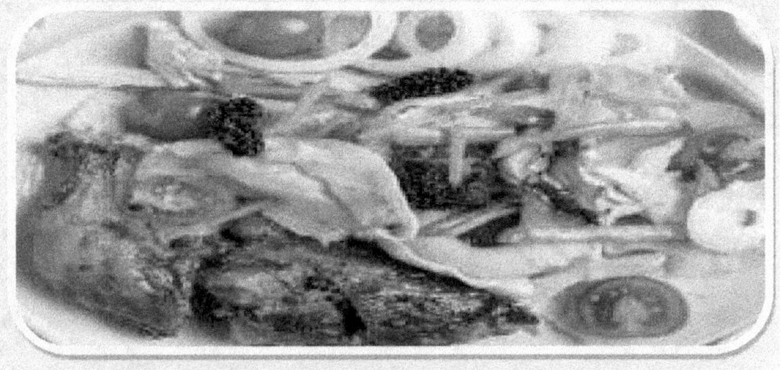

Gestational Recipes for dinner

Grilled lemon-herb chicken

INGREDIENTS

- 4 skinless, boneless breasts of chicken
- Olive oil, two tablespoons
- Juiced and zested one lemon
- 2 minced garlic cloves
- 1 tablespoon chopped fresh rosemary
- pepper and salt as desired–

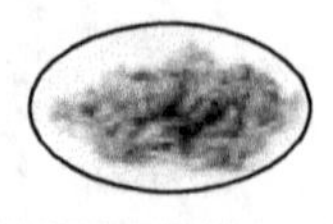 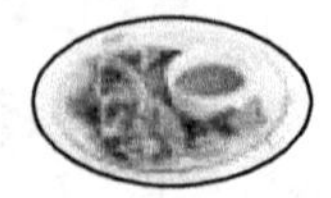 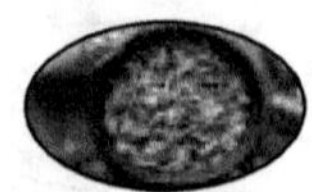

Olive oil, lemon juice, lemon zest, garlic, and rosemary should all be combined in a bowl.

Chicken breasts should be marinated in the marinade for 30 minutes.

Heat the grill to medium-high.

Cook the chicken thoroughly on the grill for 6 to 8 minutes on each side.

salt and pepper should be added to taste.

VALUE NUTRITIVE (PER SERVING):

220 calories

30g of protein

2g of carbohydrates

0g of fiber

20 minutes for cooking–

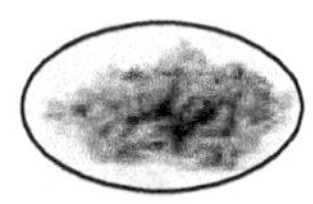 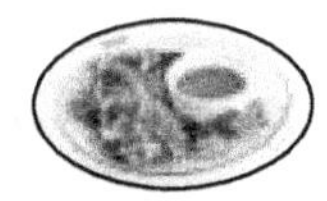 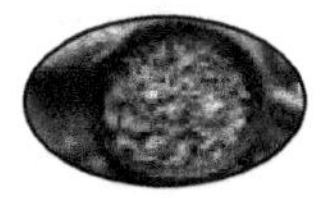

Quinoa and black bean salad

INGREDIENTS:

- quinoa, one cup
- 1 can (15 oz) washed and drained black beans
- 1 cup halved cherry tomatoes
- Diced red bell pepper(Half cup)
- 1/8 cup chopped fresh cilantro
- lime juice, 2 tablespoons
- Olive oil, two tablespoons
- salt and pepper should be added to your desired taste.

PREPARATION

Quinoa should be prepared as directed on the packaging.

Quinoa, black beans, cherry tomatoes, red bell pepper, and cilantro should all be combined in a big bowl.

Mix the lime juice, olive oil, salt, and pepper in a another bowl.

Mix the salad after adding the dressing.–

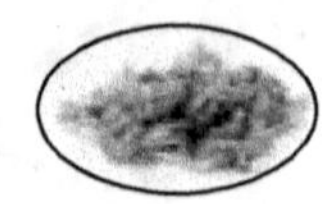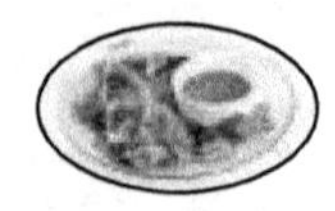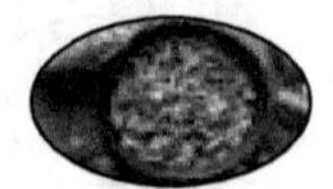

250 calories

8g protein

38g of carbohydrates

6g of fiber

Preparation Time: 25 minutes

Salmon and asparagus baked

INGREDIENTS:

- 4 fillets of salmon
- 2 spears of asparagus
- Olive oil, two tablespoons
- 1 sliced lemon
- 2 minced garlic cloves
- one tablespoon of dried dill
- pepper and salt as desired

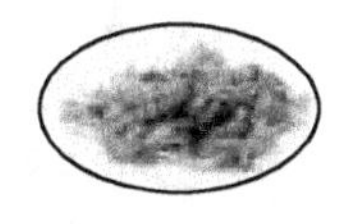 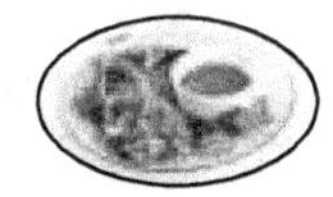 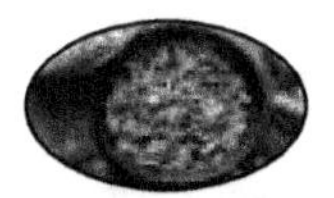

Oven should be heated to 375°F (190°C).

Insert the Salmon fillets on the baking pan.

Around the fish, arrange the asparagus.

Add garlic, dill, salt, and pepper after drizzling olive oil over the fish and asparagus.

Slices of lemon should be added.

Salmon should easily flake after baking for 15 to 20 minutes.

Value nutritive (per serving):

320 calories

30g of protein

8g of carbohydrates

3g of fiber

Preparation Time: 25 minutes–

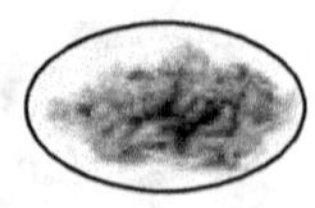 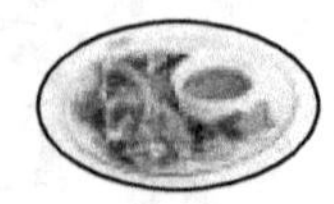 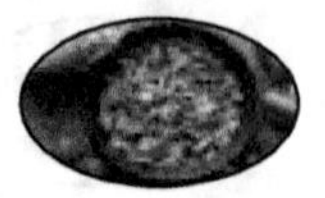

Chicken Stuffed with Spinach and Mushrooms

INGREDIENTS:

- 4 skinless, boneless breasts of chicken
- Fresh spinach, 2 cups
- 1 cup of sliced mushrooms
- low-fat mozzarella cheese, 1/4 cup
- 2 minced garlic cloves
- 1/9 cup olive oil
- pepper and salt as desired

PREPARATION:

Oven should be heated to 375°F (190°C).

Sauté mushrooms and garlic in oil in a pan until they are tender.

After adding, boil spinach until wilted.

Indent each chicken breast with a pocket.

Place the mixture of spinach and mushrooms within, and top with mozzarella cheese.

Bake the chicken for 25 to 30 minutes, or until done.–

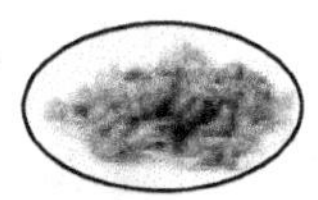 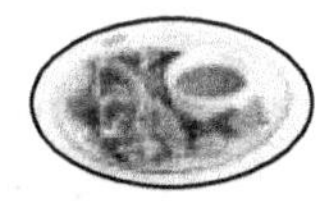 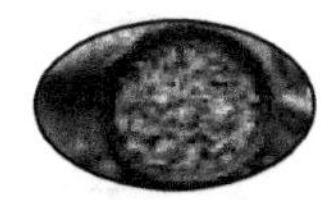

Value nutritive (per serving):

280 calories

40g of protein

4g of carbohydrates

2g of fiber

35 minutes for cooking

Lentil and vegetable curry

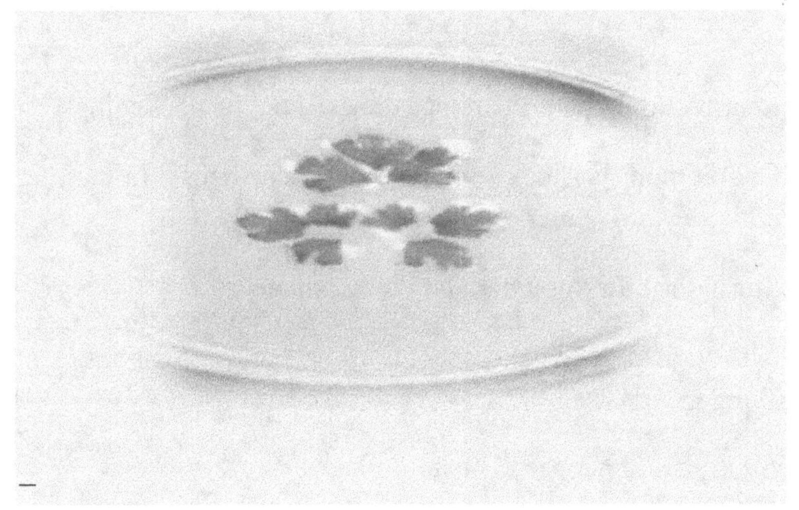

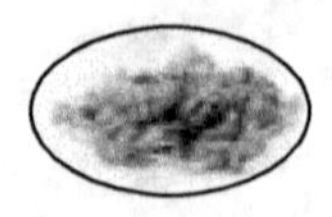 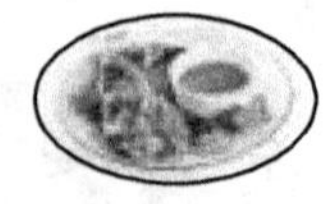 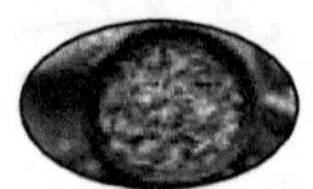

INGREDIENTS:

- Dried green lentils, 1 cup
- one sliced onion
- 2 minced garlic cloves
- one carrot, diced
- 1 chopped bell pepper
- 1 can (14 oz) shredded tomatoes
- Curry powder, two tablespoons
- 1 can (14 oz) coconut cream
- pepper and salt as desired

PREPARATION:

Lentils should be prepared as directed on the packaging.

Cook onion, garlic, carrot, and bell pepper in a big skillet until they are tender.

Stir in the curry powder and diced tomatoes.

Add cooked lentils and coconut milk. For 15 to 20 minutes, simmer.

Add salt and pepper to taste.–

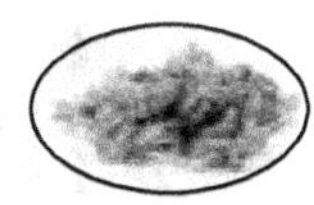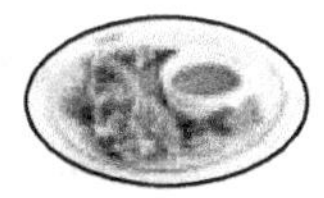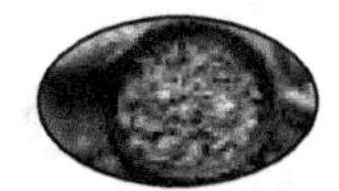

Value nutritive (per serving):

350 calories

15g of protein

45g of carbohydrates

14g of fiber

Preparation Time: 40 minutes

Stir-fried turkey with vegetables

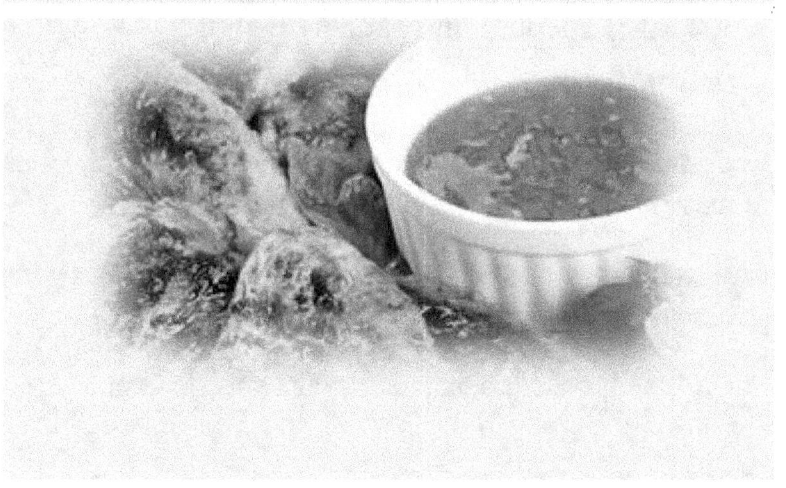

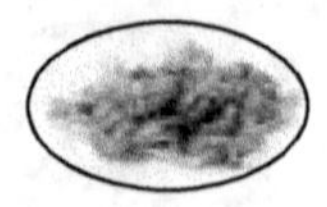 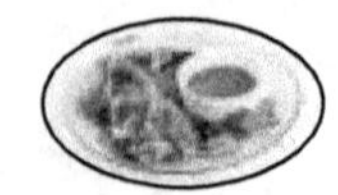 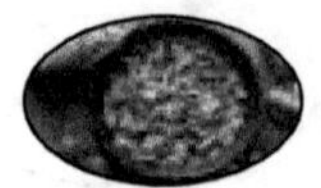

- 1 pound of turkey meat
- 200 grams of broccoli florets
- 1 cup thinly chopped bell peppers
- Snap peas, 1 cup
- Low-sodium soy sauce, two tablespoons
- one teaspoon of sesame oil
- 1 teaspoon of minced ginger
- 2 minced garlic cloves
- pepper and salt as desired

PREPARATION:

Cook ground turkey till browned in a large skillet. Exit it out of the skillet and place in a different place.

Garlic and ginger should be cooked in the same skillet with sesame oil until aromatic.

Stir-fry the broccoli, bell peppers, and snap peas until they are soft.

Soy sauce is added to the skillet with the turkey and is cooked for an additional two to three minutes.

Add salt and pepper to taste.–

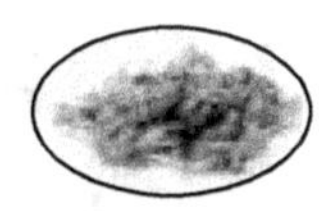 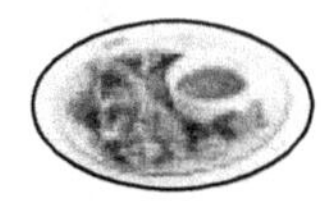 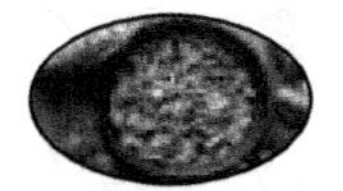

Value nutritive (per serving):

290 calories

25g of protein

15g of carbohydrates

5g of fiber

Preparation Time: 25 minutes

Pesto-topped Zucchini Noodles

INGREDIENTS:

- (Noodles made from spiralized four medium zucchini)
- a half-cup of basil pesto sauce
- grated Parmesan cheese, 1/4 cup
- cherry tomatoes as an ornament
- pepper and salt as desired

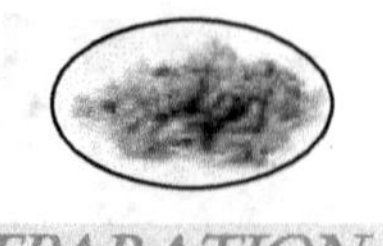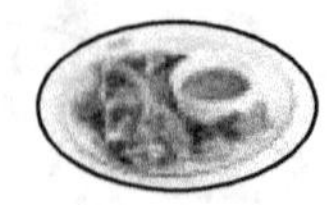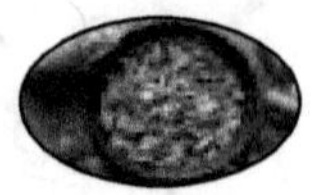

Make zucchini noodles by spiralizing them.

Zucchini noodles should be heated through in a big pan.

Add grated Parmesan cheese and pesto sauce before tossing.

Add cherry tomatoes as a garnish.

Add salt and pepper to taste.

Value nutritive (per serving):

220 calories

5g protein

10g of carbohydrates

3g of fiber

15 minutes for cooking–

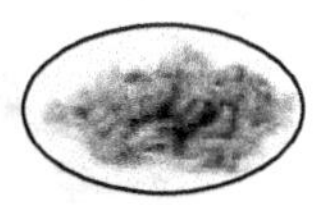 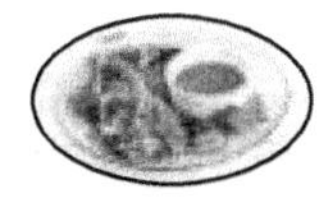 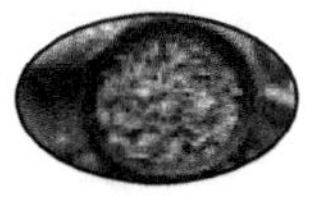

Sweet potato and black bean enchiladas (baked)

INGREDIENTS:

- Four little sweet potatoes
- 1 can (15 oz) washed and drained black beans
- One salsa cup
- 1 cup of cheddar cheese, shredded
- Eight tiny whole-wheat tortillas
- Pepper and salt as desired

PREPARATION:

Oven should be heated to 375°F (190°C).

Sweet potatoes should be baked for 45 minutes or until soft.

Remove the flesh, then mash it with salsa, black beans, salt, and pepper.

The sweet potato mixture should be rolled up within tortillas, then placed in a baking dish.

Shredded cheese should melt and bubble after 20 to 25 minutes in the oven.

Value nutritive (per serving):

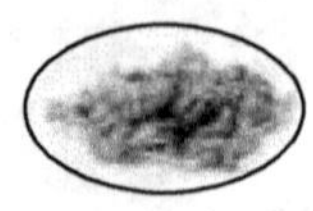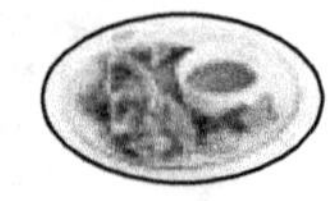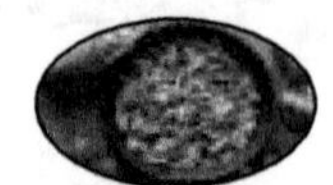

380 calories

14g of protein

60g of carbohydrates

12g of fiber

Preparation Time: 75 minutes

Cod baked in a lemon-dill sauce

INGREDIENTS:

4 fillets of cod

Olive oil, two tablespoons

two teaspoons of lemon juice, fresh

1 teaspoon chopped fresh dill

2 minced garlic cloves

pepper and salt as desired–

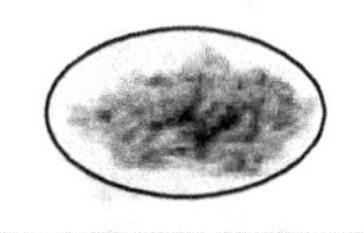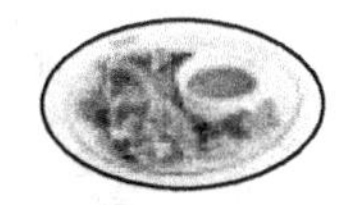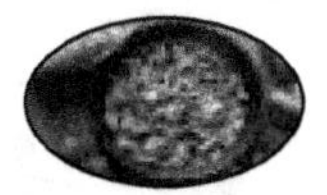

Oven should be heated to 375°F (190°C).

Cod fillets must be inserted on a baking dish.

Mix the olive oil, lemon juice, dill, garlic, salt, and pepper in a small bowl.

Bake the fish for fifteen minutes.

Value nutritive (per serving):

190 calories

26g of protein

2g of carbohydrates

0g of fiber

Preparation Time: 25 minutes–

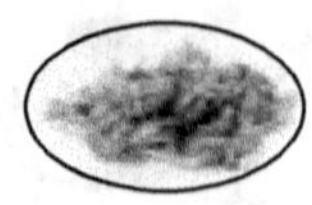 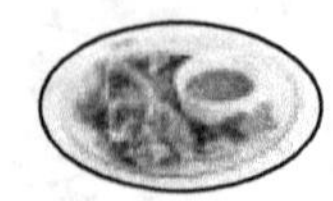 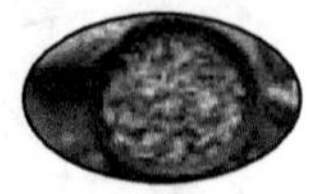

Stir-fried vegetables and tofu

INGREDIENTS:

- 1 cubed block of tofu
- 2 cups of mixed vegetables (carrots, snap peas, bell peppers, broccoli)
- Low-sodium soy sauce, two tablespoons
- one teaspoon of sesame oil
- 1 teaspoon of minced ginger
- 2 minced garlic cloves
- salt and pepper must be added to taste.

PREPARATION

Garlic and ginger should be cooked in sesame oil until aromatic.

Tofu cubes should be added and stir-fried until just faintly browned.

After adding the mixed vegetables, stir-fry them further until they are soft.

Add the soy sauce, then simmer for an additional two to three minutes.

Add salt and pepper to taste.

Value nutritive (per serving):–

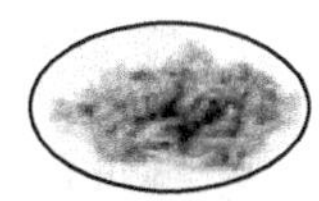 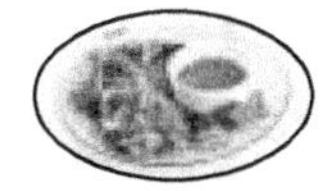 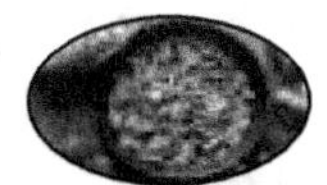

280 calories

18g of protein

15g of carbohydrates

4g of fiber

Preparation Time: 25 minutes

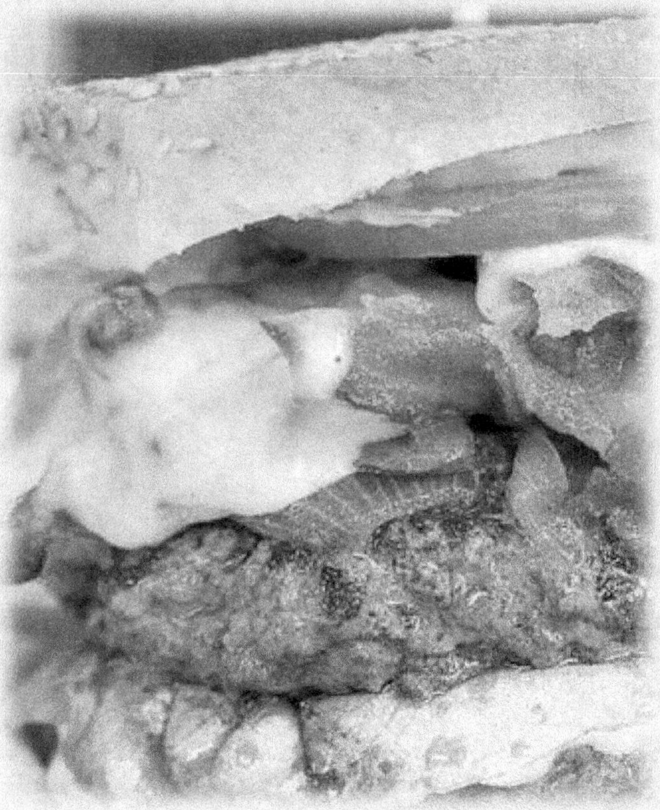

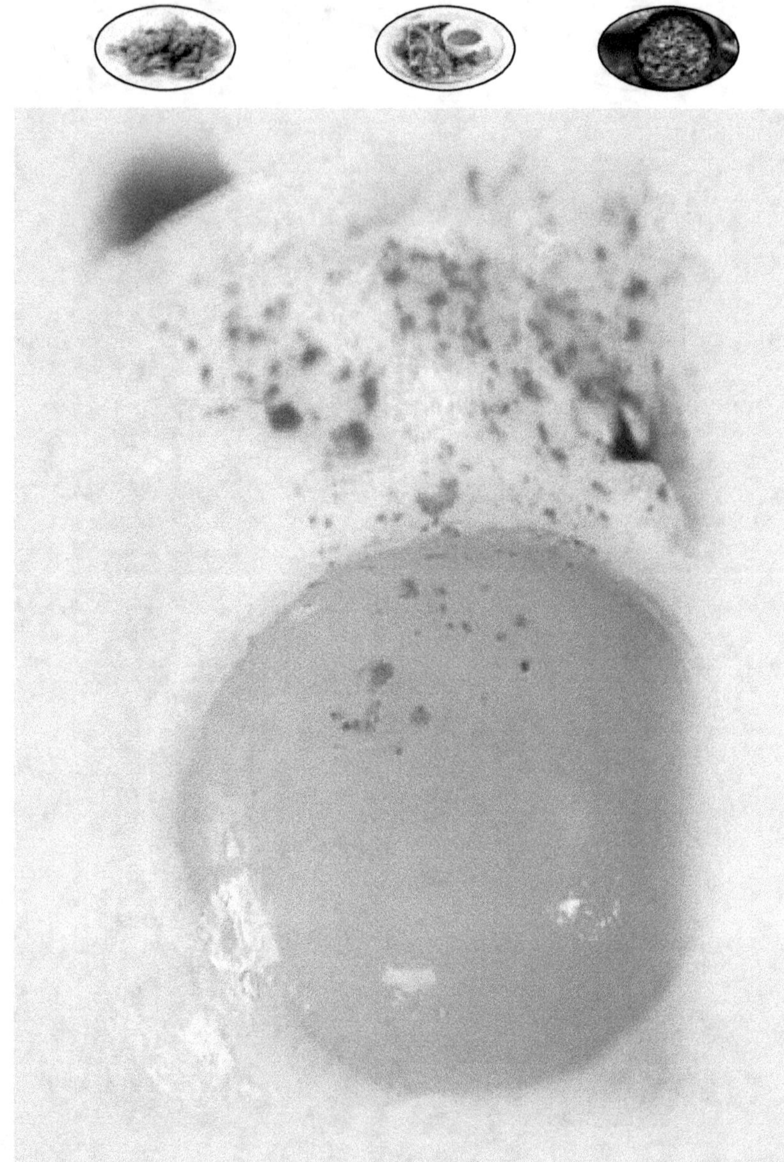

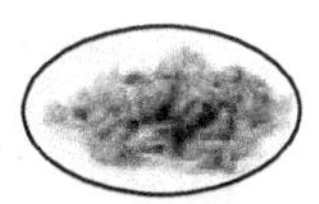 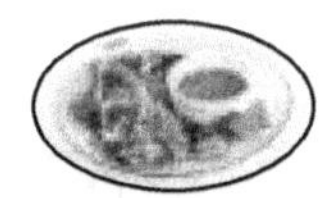 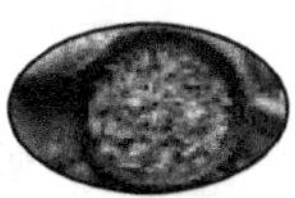

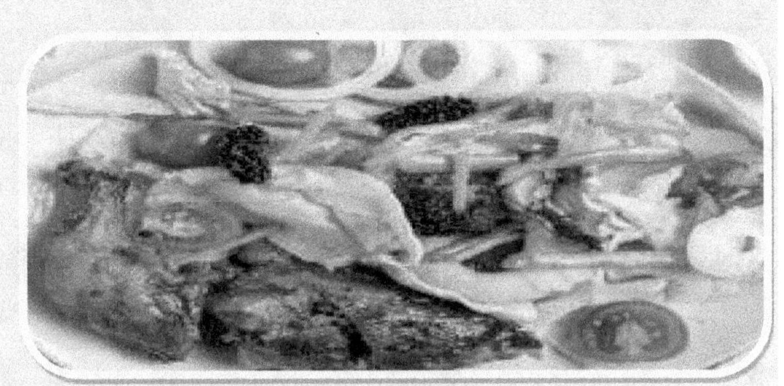

Snacks and little meals

Greek yogurt and cucumber dip

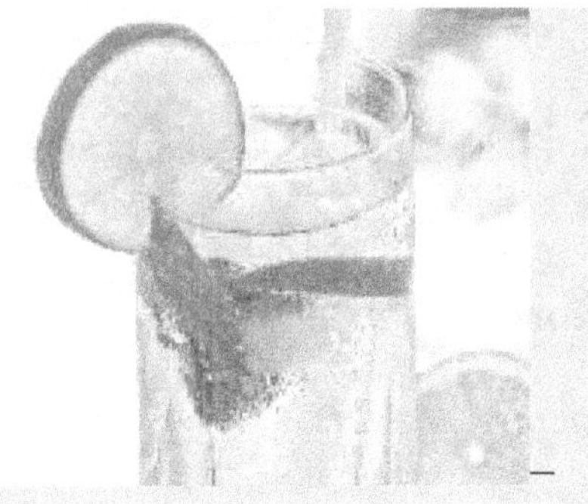

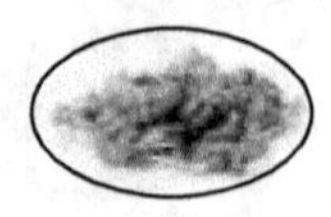 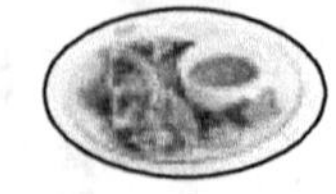 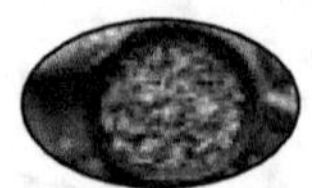

INGREDIENTS:

Grated one medium cucumber, one cup of basic Greek yogurt

1 minced garlic clove

1 tablespoon finely chopped fresh dill Salt and pepper as desired

NUTRITIVE WORTH:

85 calories

8g of carbohydrates

10g of protein

1g of fiber

PREPARATION:

Grate the cucumber, then press off any extra liquid.

Grated cucumber, Greek yogurt, minced garlic, and fresh dill should all be combined in a bowl.

Add salt and pepper to taste.

Prior to serving with sliced vegetables, chill in the refrigerator for at least 30 minutes.–

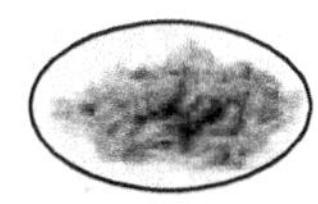 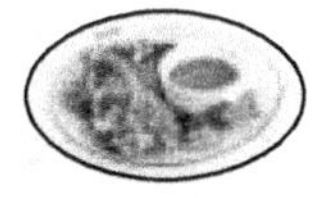 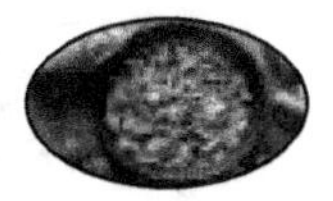

Berry and Almond Energy Bites

INGREDIENTS:

- 1 cup of ground almonds
- Cranberries, blueberries, or strawberries make up half a cup of dried berries.
- quarter cup of almond butter
- Honey, 1/4 cup
- One-half teaspoon of vanilla extract

NUTRITIVE WORTH:

120 calories

11g of carbohydrates

3g. protein

2g of fiber

PREPARATION:

Almonds and dried berries should be processed in a food processor to a fine powder.

Add vanilla essence, honey, and almond butter. Once everything is thoroughly blended, pulse.

Make bite-sized balls out of the mixture.–

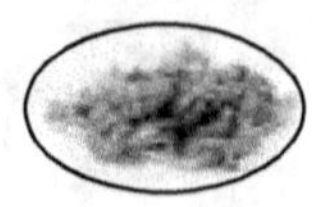 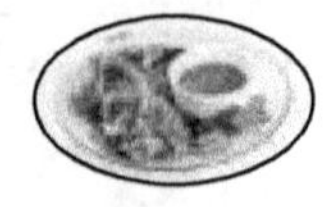 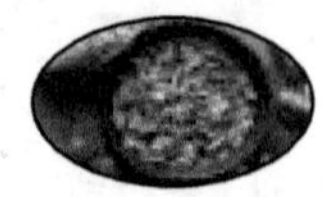

Refrigerate for atleast 30 minutes before serving

Tomato-Avocado Salsa

INGREDIENTS:

2 ripe avocados, diced; 2 medium tomatoes, diced; 1/4 cup finely chopped red onion; 1/4 cup chopped fresh cilantro; and 1 lime juice.

Pepper and salt as desired

NUTRITIVE WORTH:

120 calories

8g of carbohydrates

2g protein

5g of fiber

PREPARATION:

Avocado, tomato, red onion, and cilantro, all diced, should be combined in a bowl.

Add salt and pepper, then drizzle with lime juice.

Serve with whole-grain crackers or vegetable sticks after gently combining.–

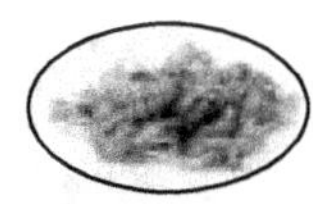 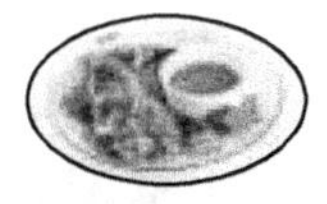 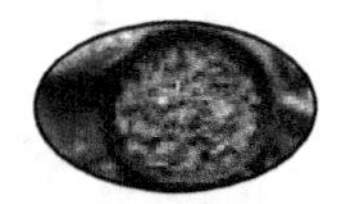

4. Stuffed peppers with cottage cheese and vegetables

- Two bell peppers should be cut in half after being seeded.
- 1 cup of cottage cheese low in fat
- Cucumber, diced, in a cup
- 1/2 cup diced bell pepper (from the tops)
- 1/4 cup red onion, chopped

Fresh herbs, such as basil or parsley, for garnish. Per stuffed pepper half, the following nutrients are provided:

90 calories

8g of carbohydrates

9g protein

2g of fiber

Preparation:

To slightly soften the bell pepper halves, steam or blanch them.

Combine cottage cheese, diced cucumber, bell pepper, and red onion in a bowl.–

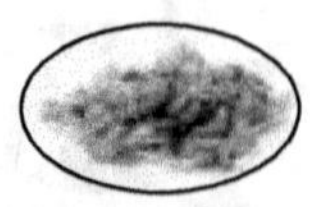 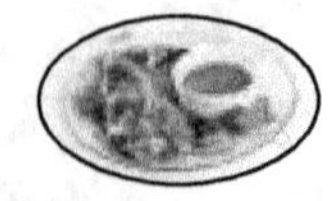 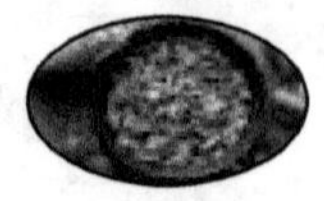

Incorporate the cottage cheese mixture into each side of the bell pepper.

Serve with fresh herbs as a garnish.

Veggie and Hummus Platter

INGREDIENTS:

50 ml of hummus

a variety of raw vegetables (cucumber, bell peppers, carrots, and celery)

NUTRITIVE WORTH:

150 calories

15g of carbohydrates

5g protein

5g of fiber

PREPARATION:

The vegetables should be washed and cut into sticks.

Serve as a dip with hummus.–

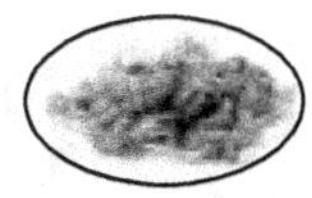 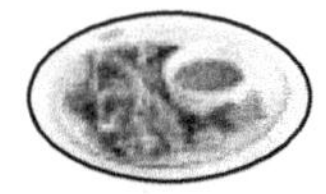 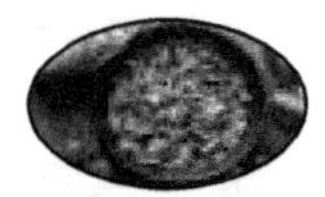

Lettuce wraps with tuna salad

INGREDIENTS:

- 1 can (5 oz) of drained tuna in water
- Greek yogurt, plain, two teaspoons
- 14 cup of celery, diced
- 1/4 cup red onion, chopped
- 1/9 cup Dijon mustard
- Leaf lettuce for wrapping

NUTRITIVE WORTH:

160 calories

3g of carbohydrates

23g of protein

1g of fiber

PREPARATION:

Tuna, Greek yogurt, celery, red onion, and Dijon mustard should all be combined in a bowl.

Wrap the tuna salad in lettuce leaves by spooning it inside.–

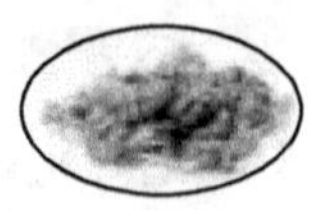 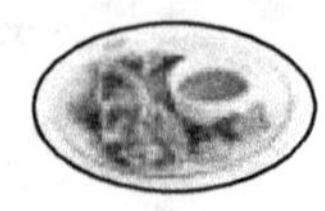 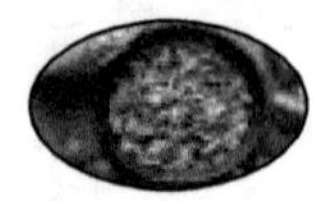

Sweet Potato Fries Baked

INGREDIENTS:

- Fries made up of two medium sweet potatoes
- Olive oil, 1 tbsp
- Paprika, half a teaspoon
- One-half teaspoon of garlic powder
- Pepper and salt as desired

NUTRITIVE WORTH:

- 120 calories
- 24g of carbohydrates
- 2g protein
- 4g of fiber

PREPARATION:

Set the oven's temperature to 425°F (220°C).

Olive oil, paprika, garlic powder, salt, and pepper are added to sweet potato fries.

Spread out on a baking sheet, then bake until crispy for 25 to 30 minutes.–

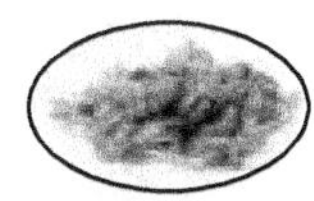 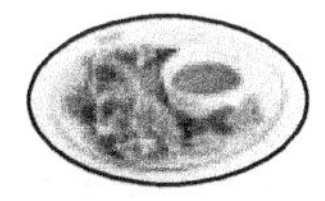 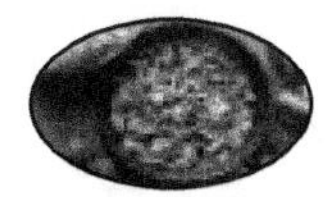

A parfait of Greek yogurt

INGREDIENTS:

1 cup of Greek yogurt, plain

14 cup of fresh berries, such as blueberries and strawberries

1 teaspoon of honey

Granola, 2 tablespoons.

NUTRITIVE WORTH:

230 calories

30g of carbohydrates

15g of protein

2g of fiber

PREPARATION:

In a glass, arrange Greek yogurt, fresh fruit, honey, and granola.

Small Caprese Skewers–

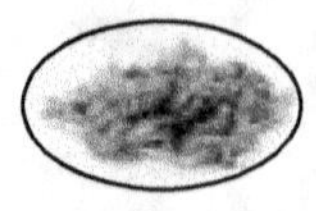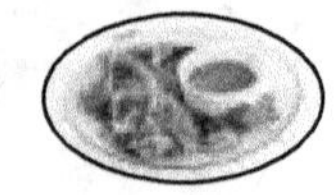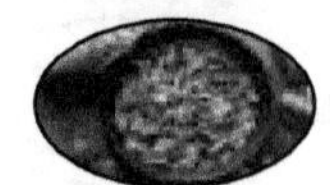

INGREDIENTS:

Plum tomatoes

balls of fresh mozzarella

fresh leaves of basil

vinegar glaze

Amount of calories in per skewer:

20 calories

2g of carbohydrates

2g protein

0g of fiber

PREPARATION:

On a toothpick, assemble a cherry tomato, a mozzarella ball, and a basil leaf.

Apply a balsamic glaze.–

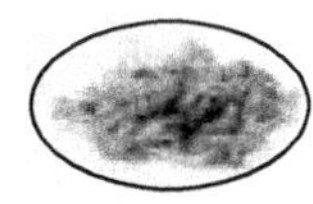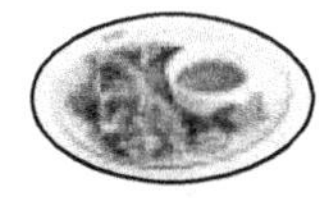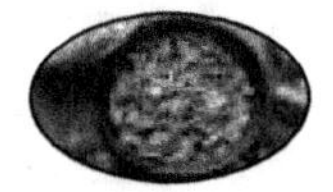

Banana slices and almond butter

INGREDIENTS:

2 tablespoons of almond butter and 1 medium banana

NUTRITIVE WORTH:

210 calories

25g of carbohydrates

5g protein

4g of fiber

PREPARATION:

Banana slices with almond butter on them should be enjoyed.

While taking into account the nutritional requirements of persons with gestational diabetes, these snacks and small nibbles offer a diversity of tastes and textures. Always keep an eye on your blood sugar levels and seek out individualized nutritional guidance from a medical practitioner.–

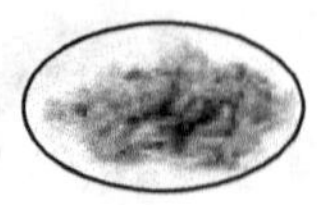 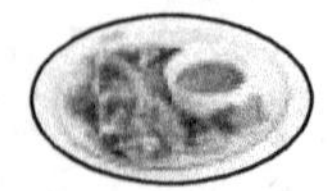 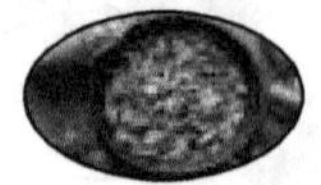

CONCLUSION

The "Gestational Diabetes Cookbook for Newly Diagnosed" is an essential tool for pregnant moms coping with the effects of gestational diabetes, to sum up. We have investigated the science behind treating this disease with food, as well as the scrumptious and nourishing options that are within our grasp.

With the knowledge and resources provided by this cookbook, newly diagnosed women are better equipped to choose a healthy diet for themselves and their unborn child. It bridges the gap between medical advice and culinary joy with healthy meal plans and delectable recipes designed for gestational diabetes.

In the course of this journey, we've discovered that managing gestational diabetes involves embracing a new way of eating that fosters wellbeing rather than depriving oneself. The given recipes have opened the door to savory and healthy meals that are tailored to the particular requirements of pregnant women.–

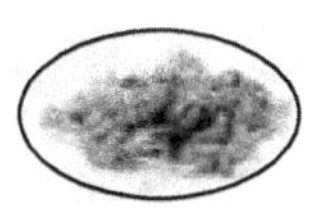 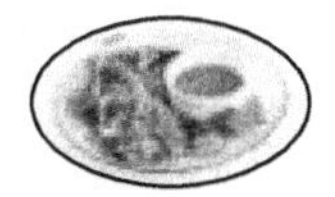 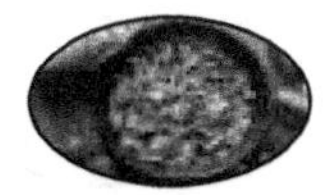

Let this cookbook serve as a ray of optimism as we draw to a close, helping you through a period of adjustment and demonstrating that gestational diabetes can be effectively and delectably managed with the correct information and a dash of creativity. May your continued journey toward a healthy pregnancy and beyond be enriched by nourishing foods and the delight of excellent health.

I appreciate your decision to buy this book despite the availability of others.

ALSO THINK ABOUT LEAVING A GOOD REVIEW SO THAT OTHERS CAN FIND THIS PRODUCT.

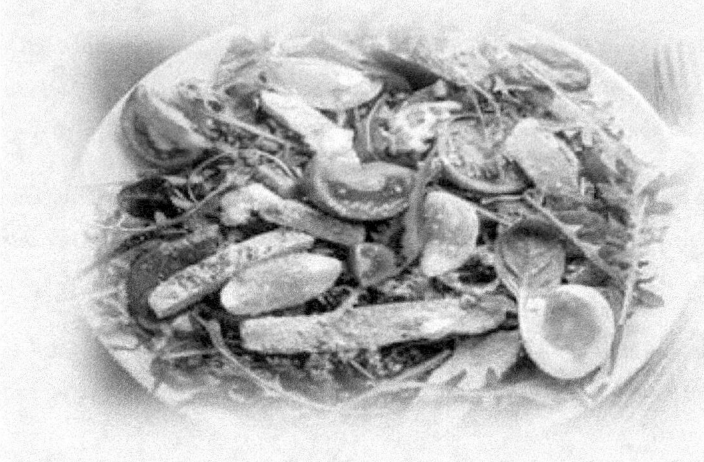

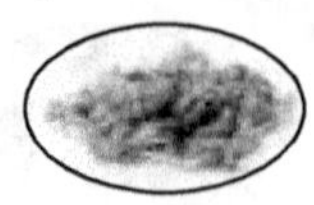 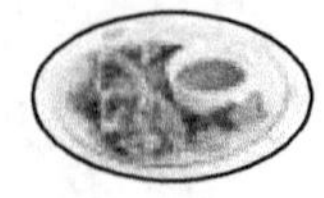 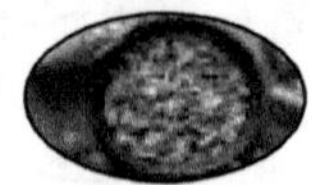

WE KNOW...

"We know time is the unit of destiny, that's why we are saying thank you."

Dear Valued Customer,

we understand that time is a precious commodity, and we sincerely appreciate you choosing to spend a portion of it with us. Your decision to trust us with your purchase means the world to us, and we want to express our deepest gratitude.

Your support not only fuels our passion for delivering quality products but also contributes to the destiny of our business. Each customer is a vital part of our journey, and we are honored to have you

We strive to provide an exceptional shopping experience, and your satisfaction is our top priority. If you have any feedback or suggestions, we would love to hear from you. Your insights help us improve.

As a small token of our appreciation, we kindly invite you to share your experience by leaving a 5-star review. Your feedback not only boosts our morale but also assists fellow shoppers in making informed decisions.

Once again, thank you for choosing to buy this book. We look forward to serving you again and being a part of your destiny in the world of quality and excellence.

Dr. Grace Hester—

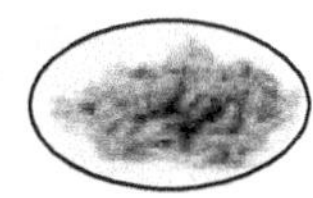 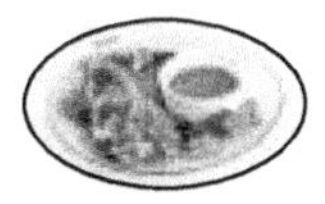 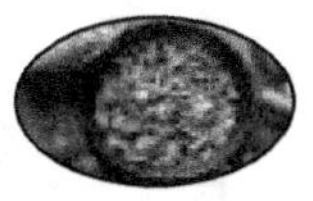

WE TRUST YOU ENJOYED THIS WONDERFUL COPY, TO ACCESS MORE BOOKS BY DR. GRACE HESTER, PROCEED TO SCAN THIS QR-CODE

–

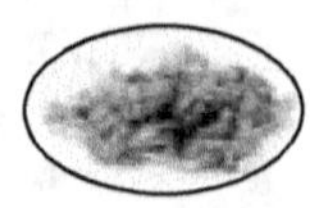 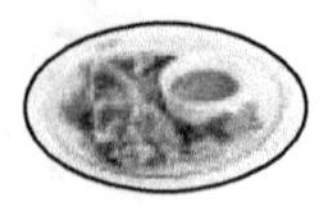 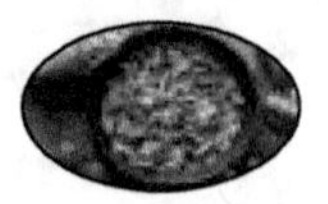

BONUS 2; MICROWAVE COOKBOOK FOR DIABETIC PATIENTS

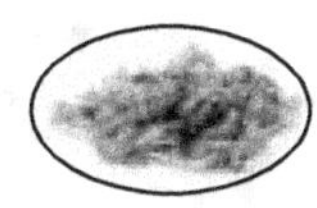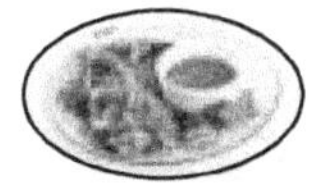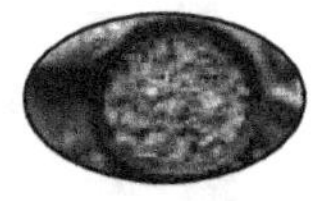

BONUS 3; DIABETES REVERSAL COOKBOOK

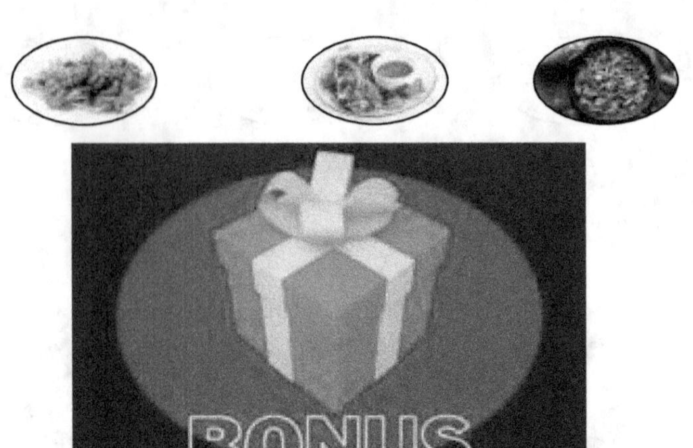

---

20 DAYS + MEAL PLANNER

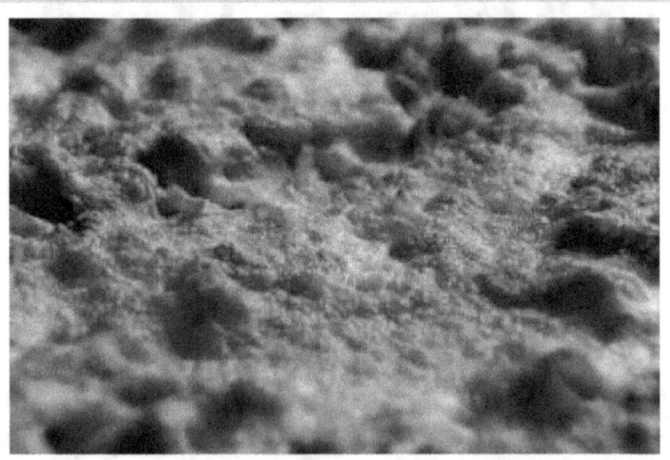

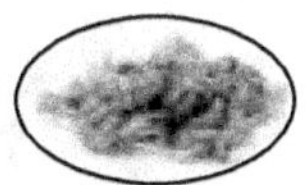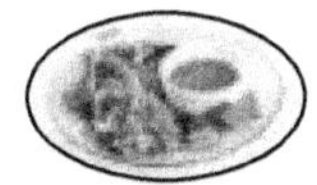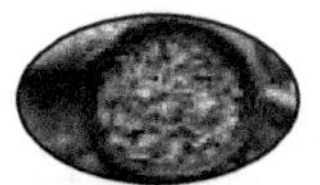

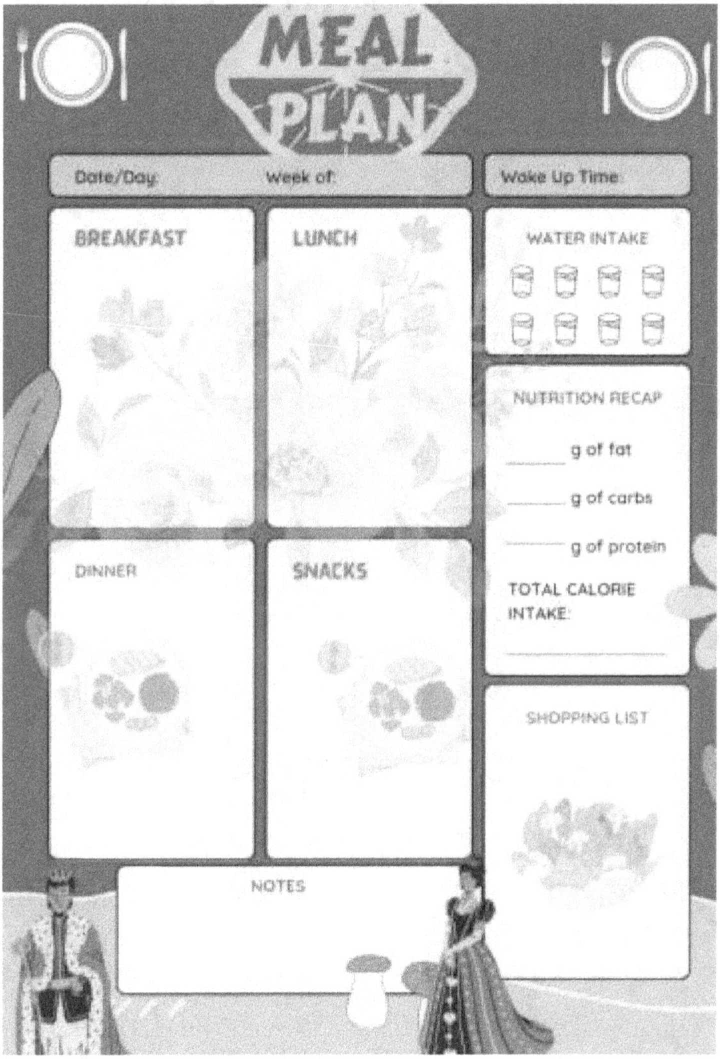

MEAL PLAN

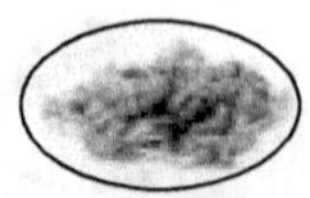 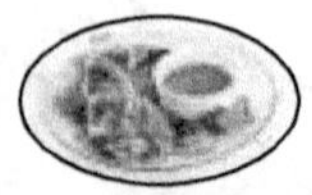 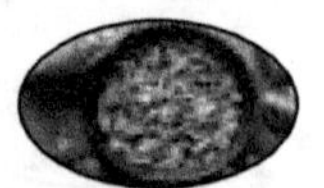

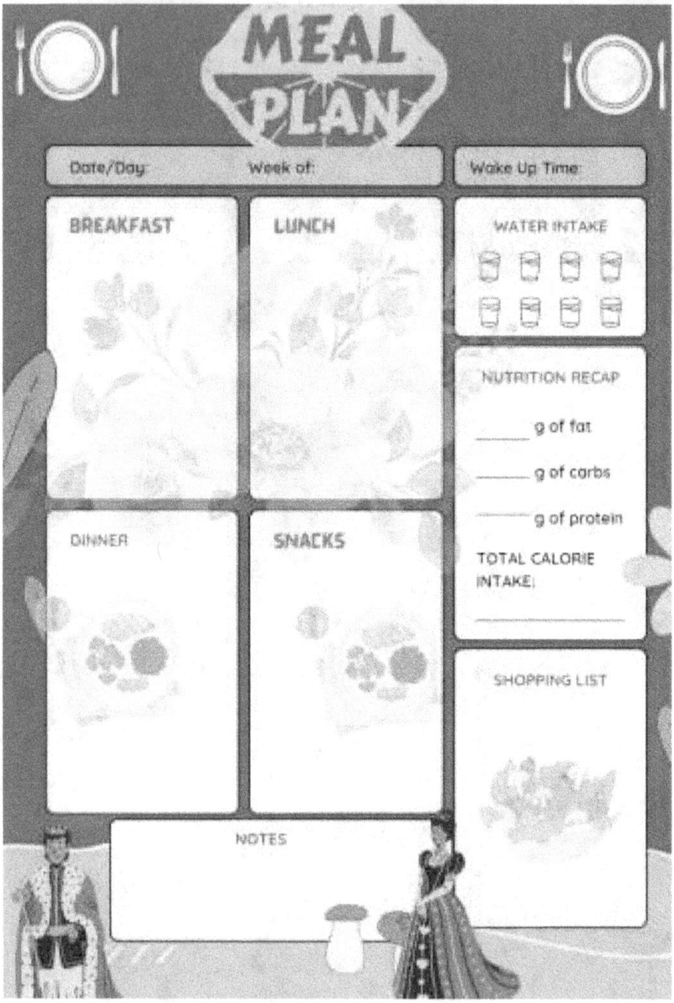

MEAL PLAN

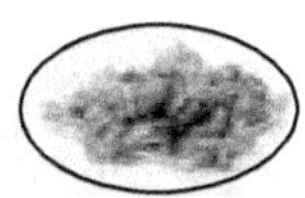 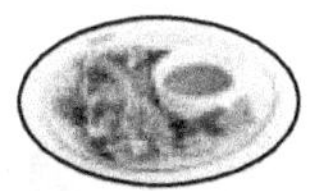 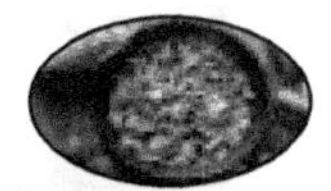

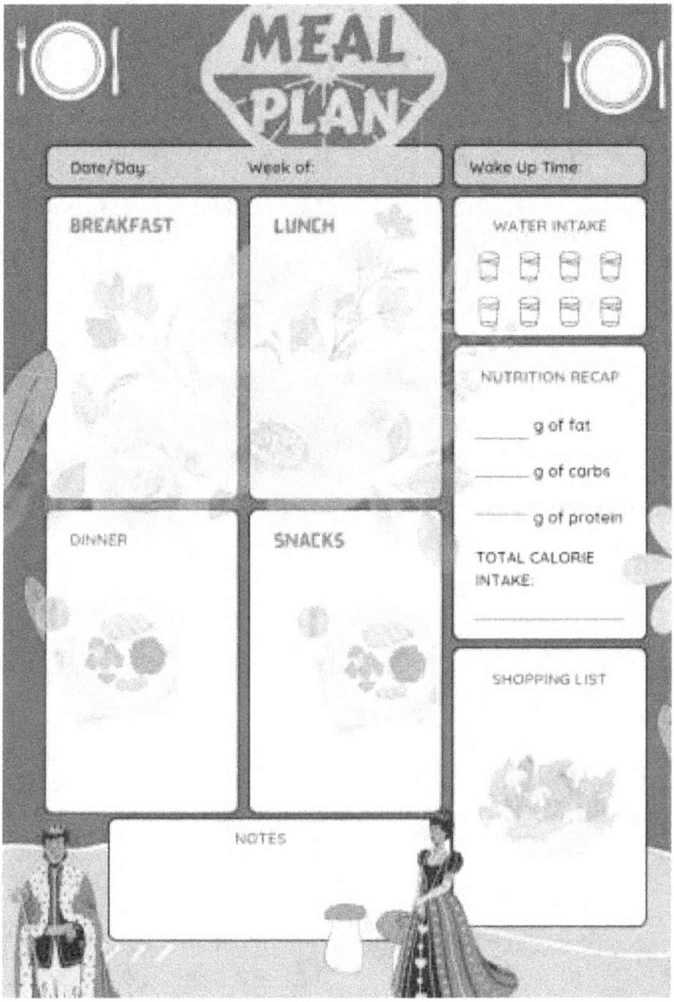

MEAL PLAN

| Date/Day | Week of: | Wake Up Time: |

BREAKFAST

LUNCH

WATER INTAKE

NUTRITION RECAP

________ g of fat

________ g of carbs

________ g of protein

TOTAL CALORIE INTAKE:

____

DINNER

SNACKS

SHOPPING LIST

NOTES

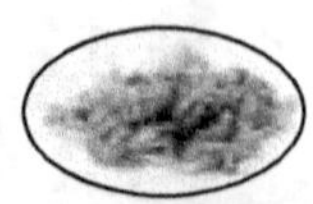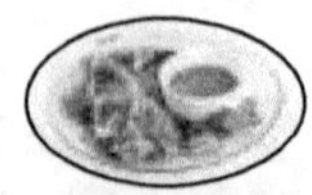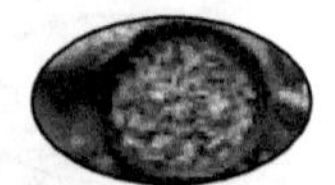

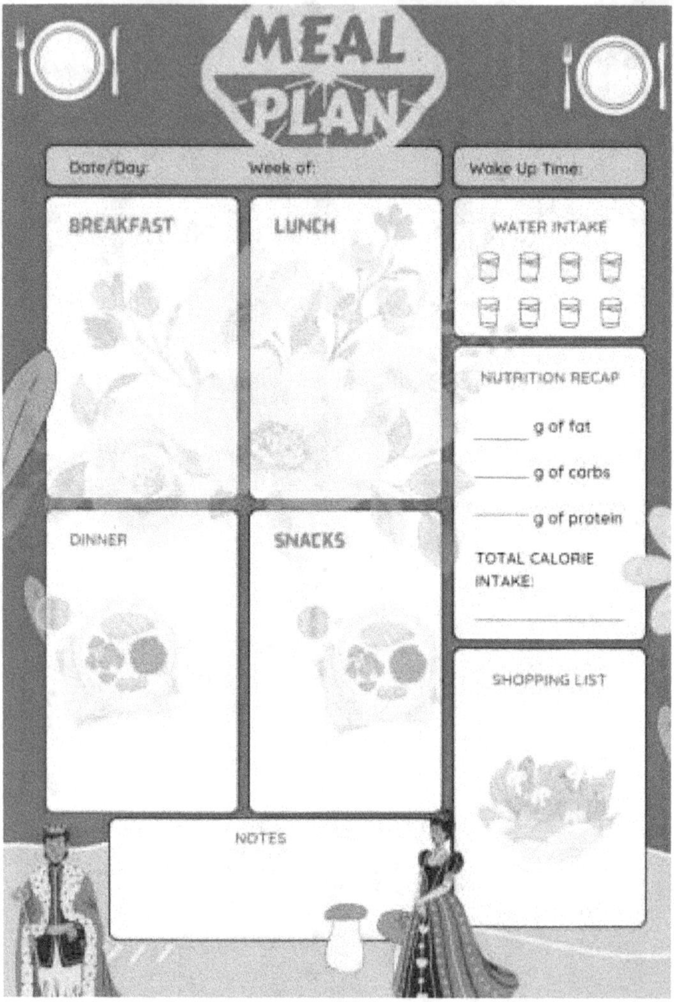

MEAL PLAN

| Date/Day: | Week of: | Wake Up Time: |

BREAKFAST

LUNCH

WATER INTAKE

NUTRITION RECAP

__________ g of fat

__________ g of carbs

__________ g of protein

TOTAL CALORIE INTAKE:

____

DINNER

SNACKS

SHOPPING LIST

NOTES

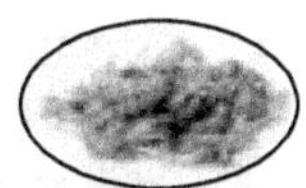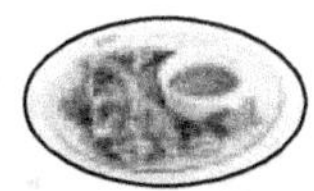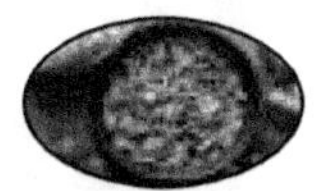

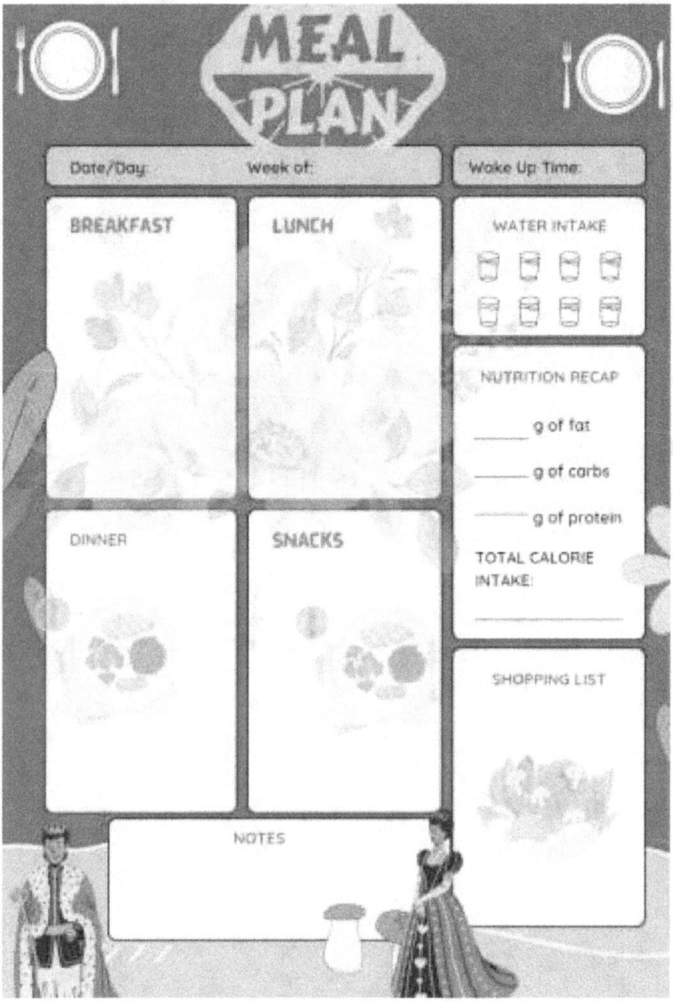

MEAL PLAN

| Date/Day | Week of: | Woke Up Time: |

BREAKFAST

LUNCH

WATER INTAKE

NUTRITION RECAP

_______ g of fat

_______ g of carbs

_______ g of protein

TOTAL CALORIE INTAKE:

____

DINNER

SNACKS

SHOPPING LIST

NOTES

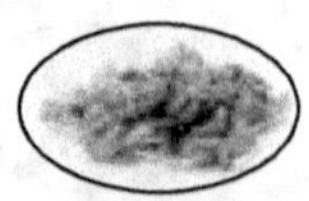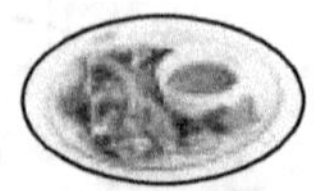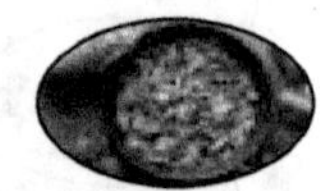

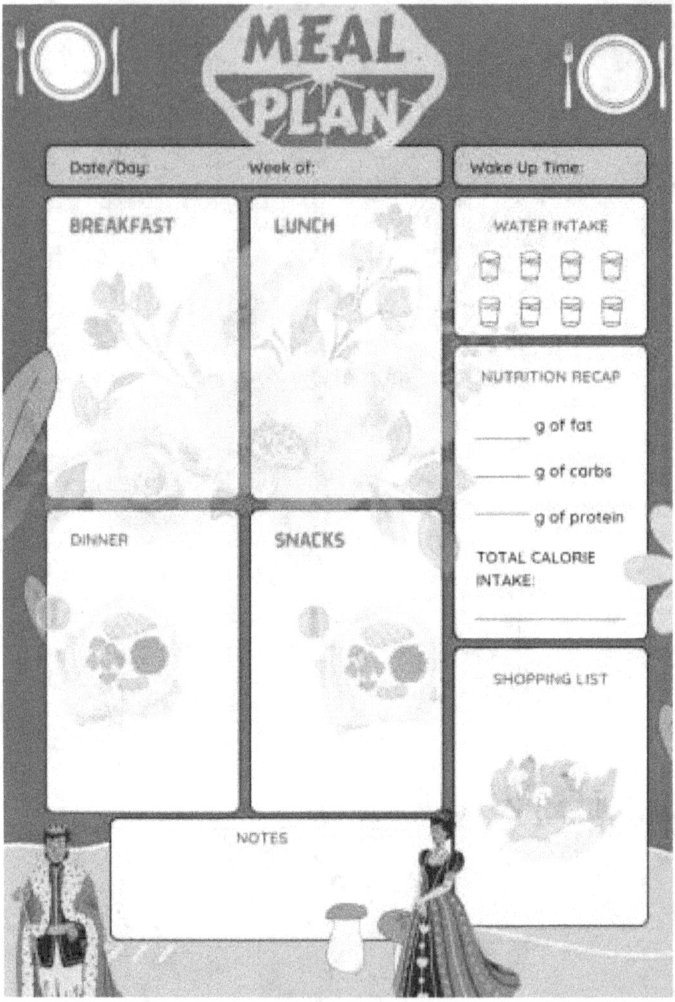

MEAL PLAN

Date/Day:	Week of:	Wake Up Time:

BREAKFAST

LUNCH

WATER INTAKE

NUTRITION RECAP

__________ g of fat

__________ g of carbs

__________ g of protein

TOTAL CALORIE INTAKE:

____

DINNER

SNACKS

SHOPPING LIST

NOTES

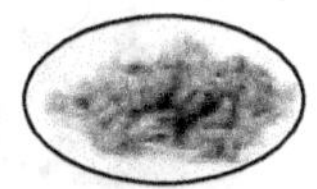 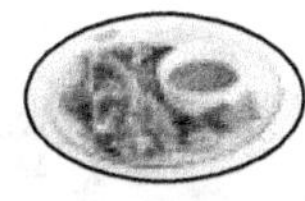 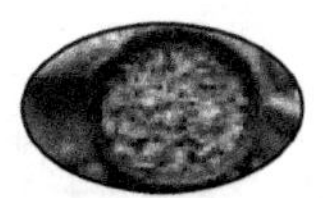

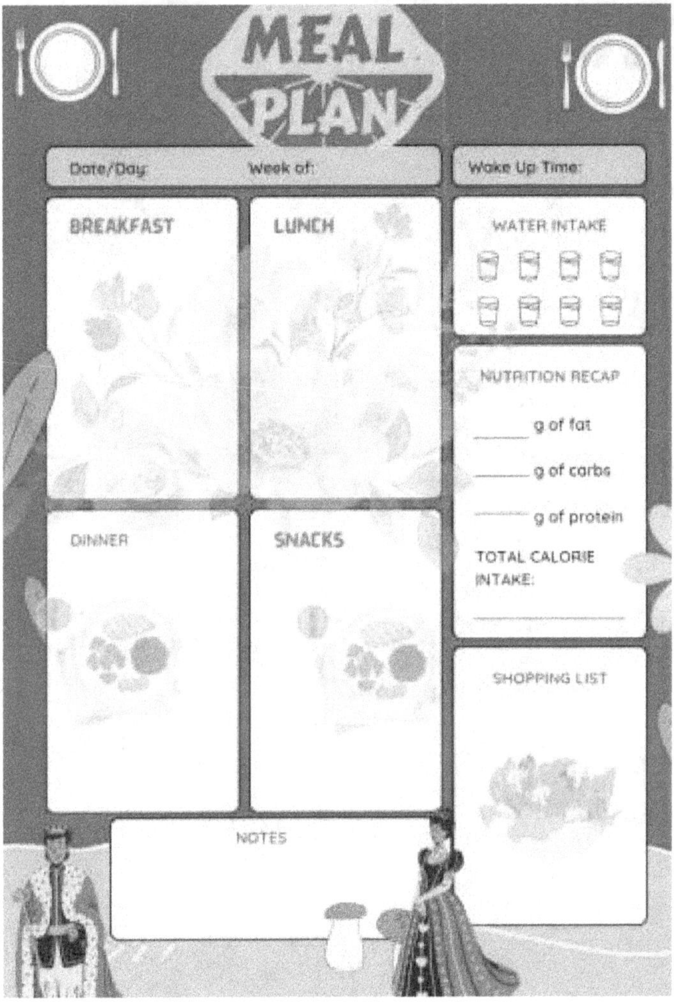

MEAL PLAN

| Date/Day | Week of: | Wake Up Time: |

BREAKFAST

LUNCH

WATER INTAKE

DINNER

SNACKS

NUTRITION RECAP

__________ g of fat

__________ g of carbs

__________ g of protein

TOTAL CALORIE INTAKE:

____

SHOPPING LIST

NOTES

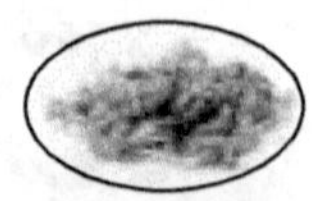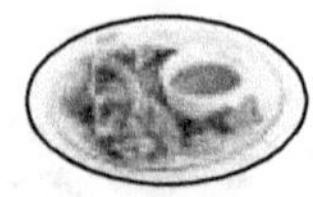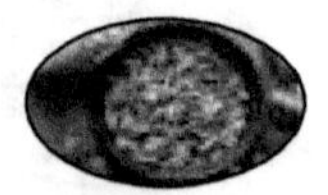

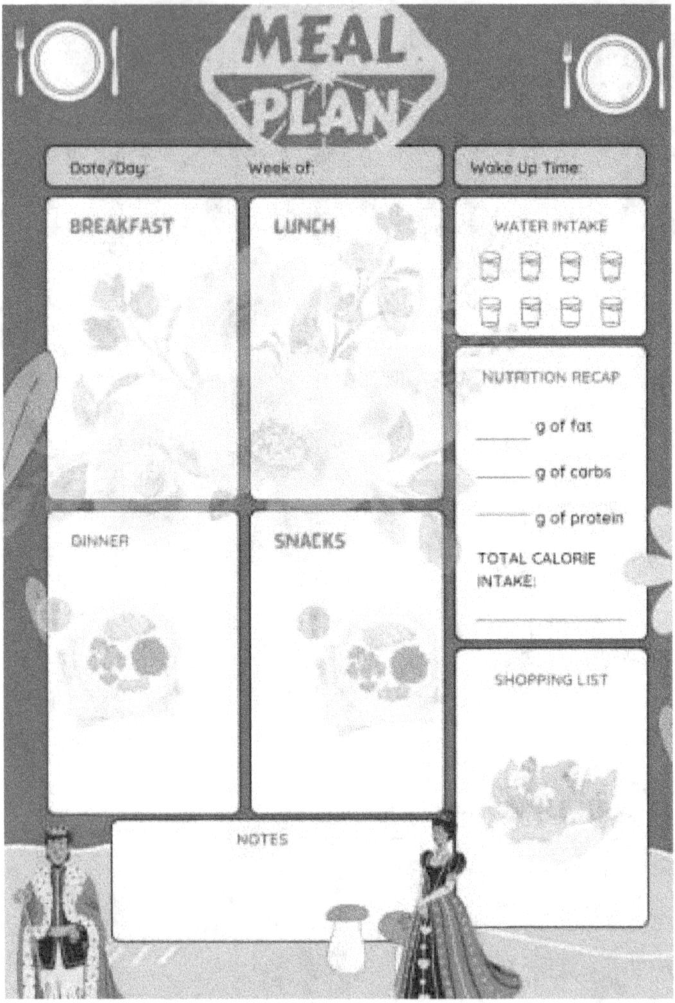

MEAL PLAN

| Date/Day: | Week of: | Wake Up Time: |

BREAKFAST

LUNCH

WATER INTAKE

NUTRITION RECAP

__________ g of fat

__________ g of carbs

__________ g of protein

TOTAL CALORIE INTAKE:

____

DINNER

SNACKS

SHOPPING LIST

NOTES

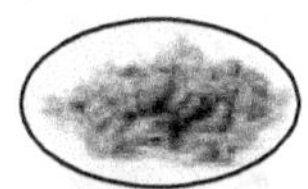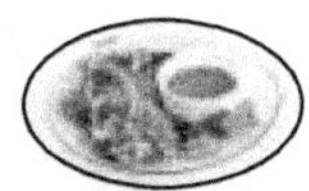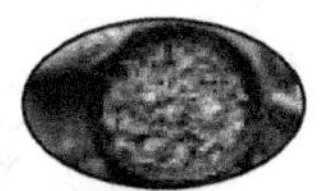

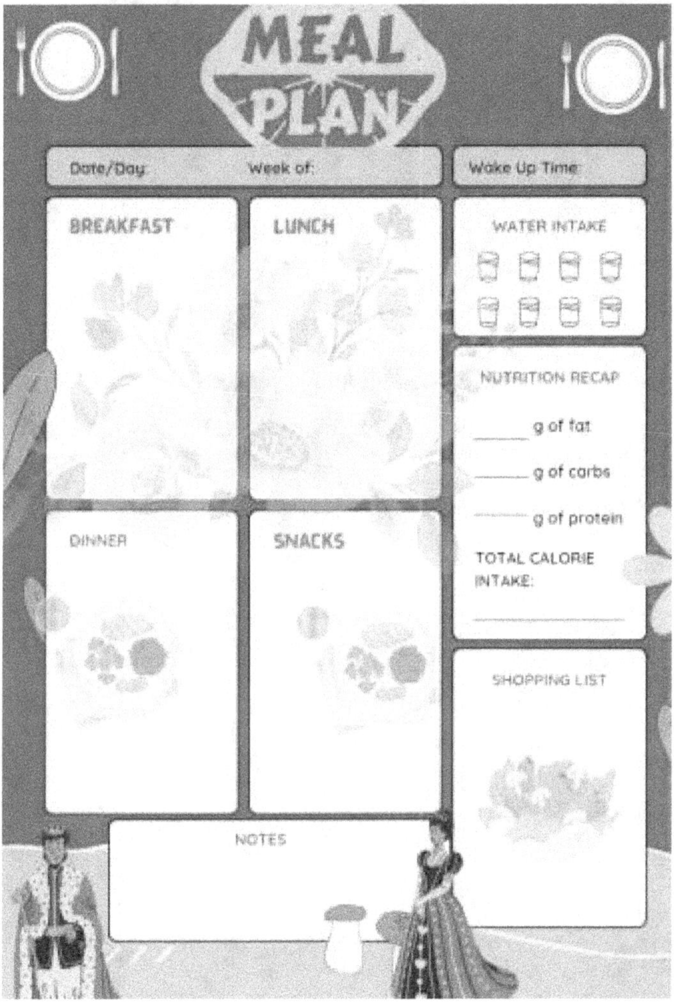

MEAL PLAN

Date/Day	Week of:	Wake Up Time:

BREAKFAST

LUNCH

WATER INTAKE

DINNER

SNACKS

NUTRITION RECAP

_______ g of fat

_______ g of carbs

_______ g of protein

TOTAL CALORIE INTAKE:

____

SHOPPING LIST

NOTES

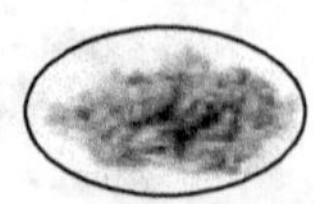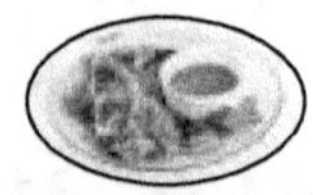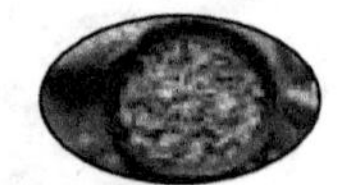

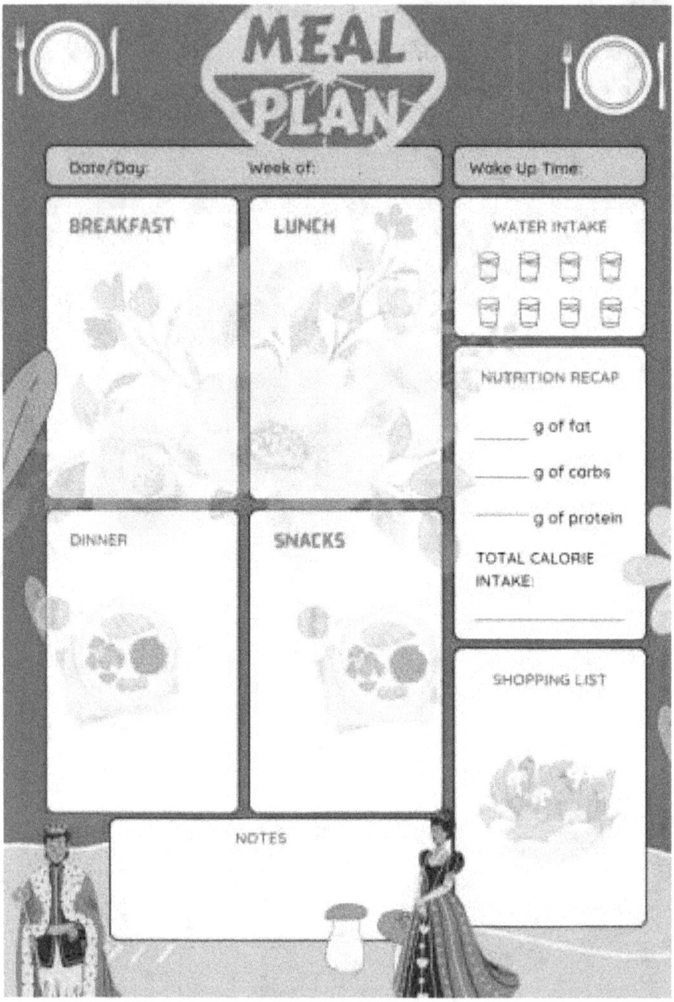

MEAL PLAN

| Date/Day: | Week of: | Wake Up Time: |

BREAKFAST

LUNCH

WATER INTAKE

NUTRITION RECAP

__________ g of fat

__________ g of carbs

__________ g of protein

TOTAL CALORIE INTAKE:

____

DINNER

SNACKS

SHOPPING LIST

NOTES

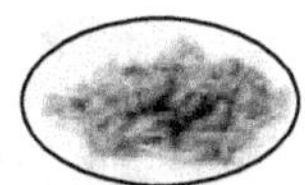
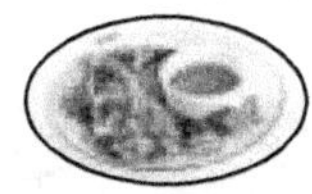
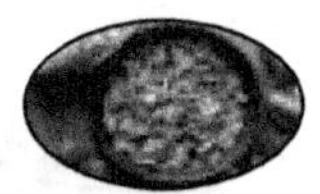

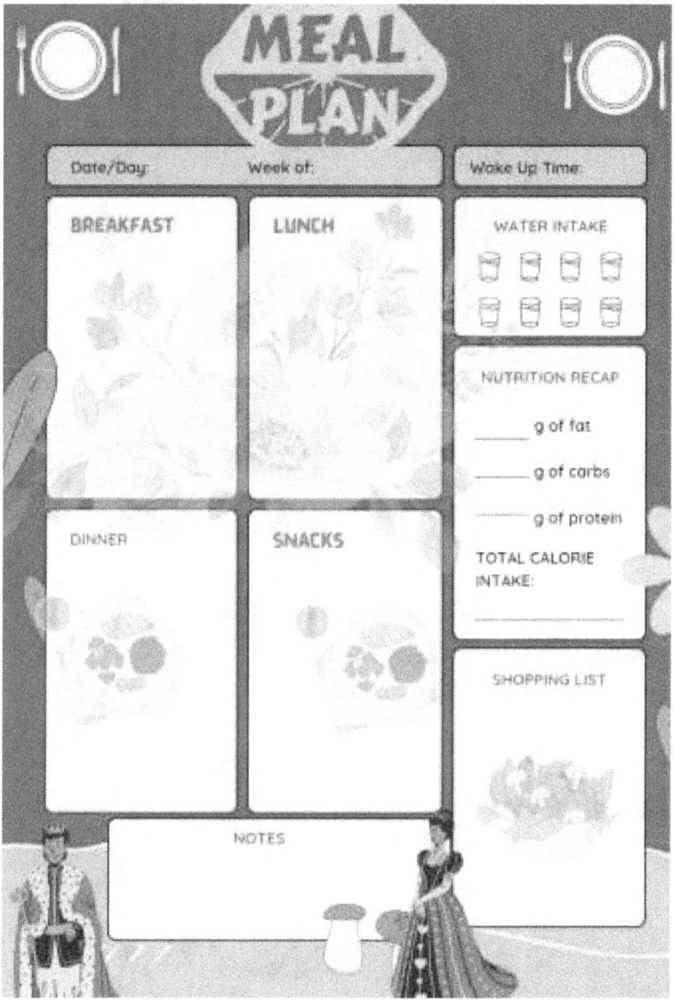

MEAL PLAN

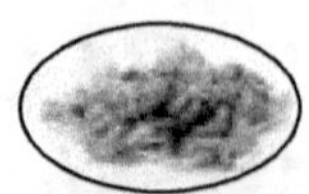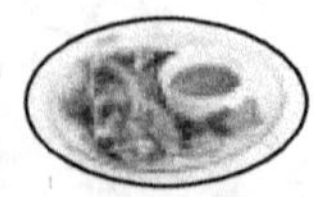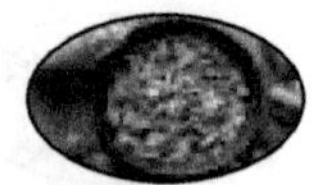

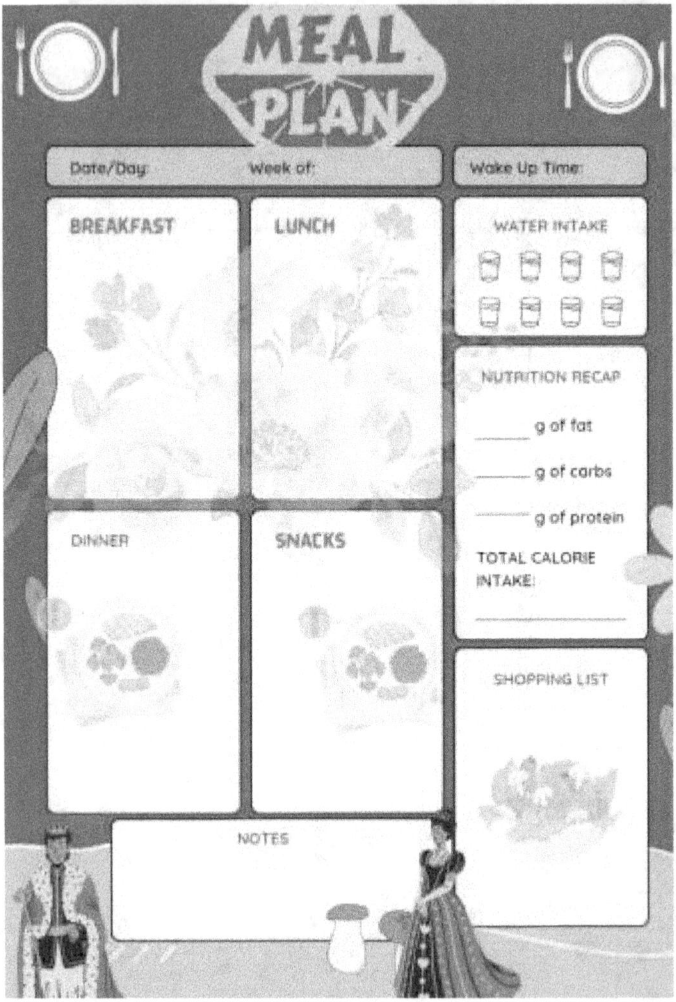

MEAL PLAN

| Date/Day: | Week of: | Wake Up Time: |

BREAKFAST

LUNCH

WATER INTAKE

NUTRITION RECAP

_______ g of fat

_______ g of carbs

_______ g of protein

TOTAL CALORIE INTAKE:

____

DINNER

SNACKS

SHOPPING LIST

NOTES

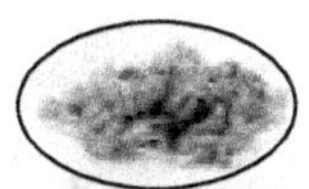 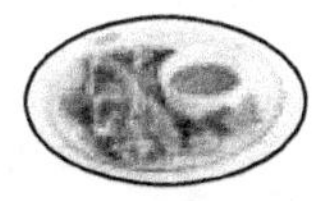 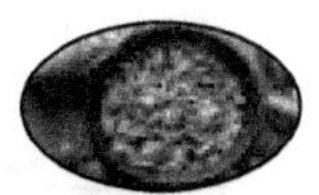

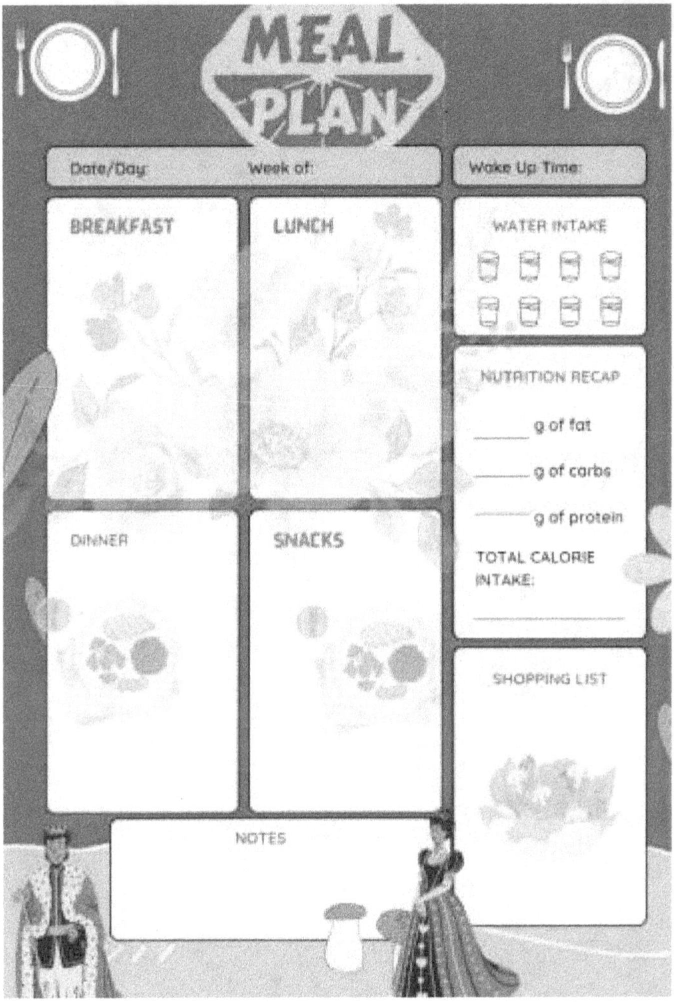

MEAL PLAN

| Date/Day: | Week of: | Wake Up Time: |

BREAKFAST

LUNCH

WATER INTAKE

NUTRITION RECAP

__________ g of fat

__________ g of carbs

__________ g of protein

TOTAL CALORIE INTAKE:

____

DINNER

SNACKS

SHOPPING LIST

NOTES

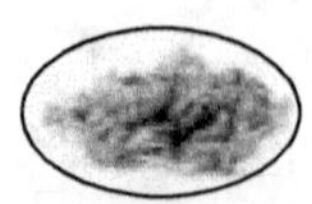 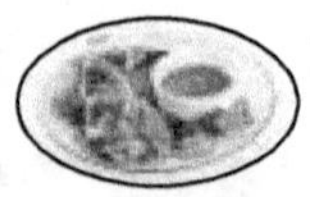 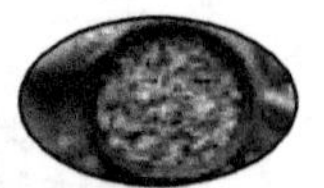

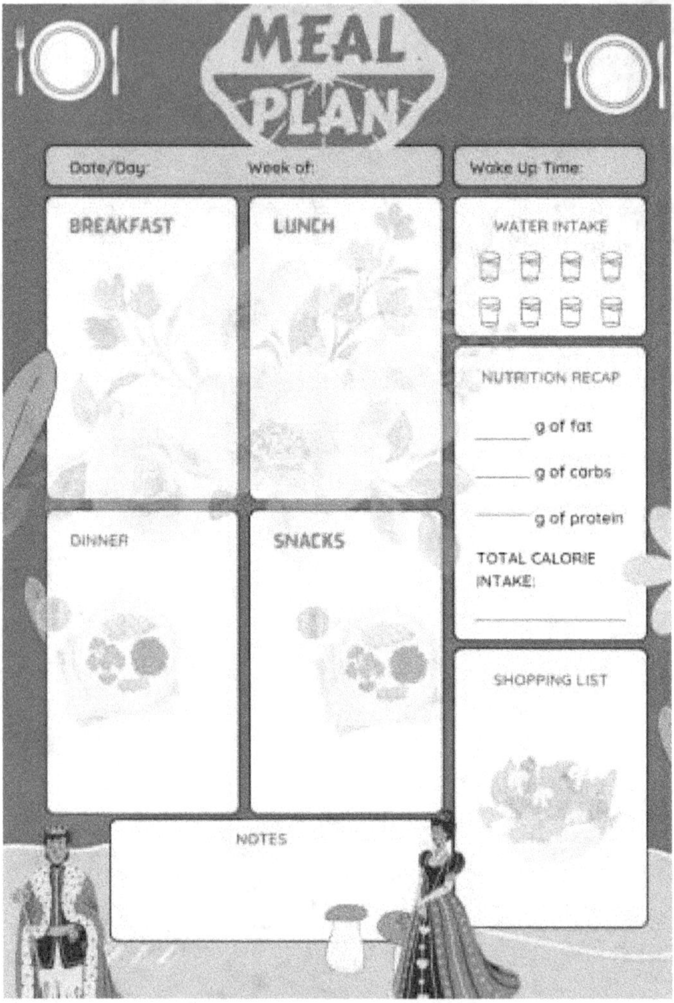

MEAL PLAN

| Date/Day: | Week of: | Wake Up Time: |

BREAKFAST

LUNCH

WATER INTAKE

NUTRITION RECAP

_______ g of fat

_______ g of carbs

_______ g of protein

TOTAL CALORIE INTAKE:

____

DINNER

SNACKS

SHOPPING LIST

NOTES

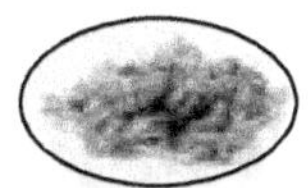
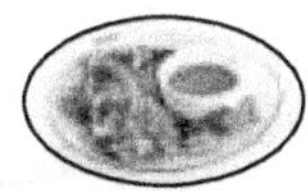
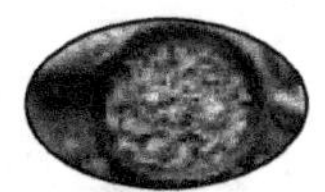

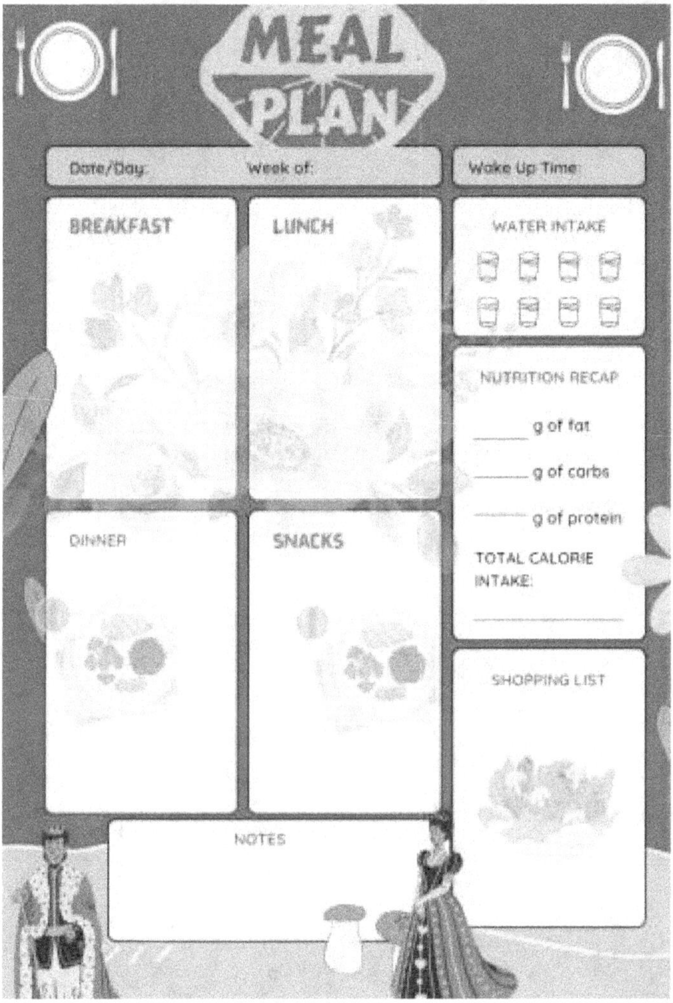

MEAL
PLAN
Date/Day: Week of:
Wake Up Time:
BREAKFAST
LUNCH
WATER INTAKE
NUTRITION RECAP
_______ g of fat
_______ g of carbs
_______ g of protein
TOTAL CALORIE
INTAKE:
DINNER
SNACKS
SHOPPING LIST
NOTES

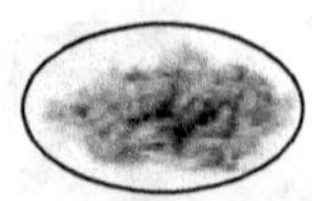 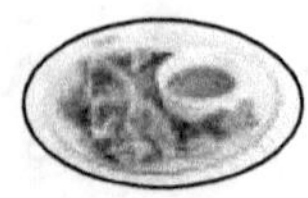 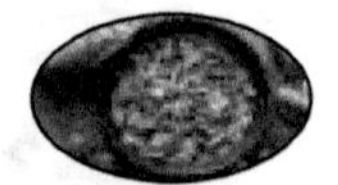

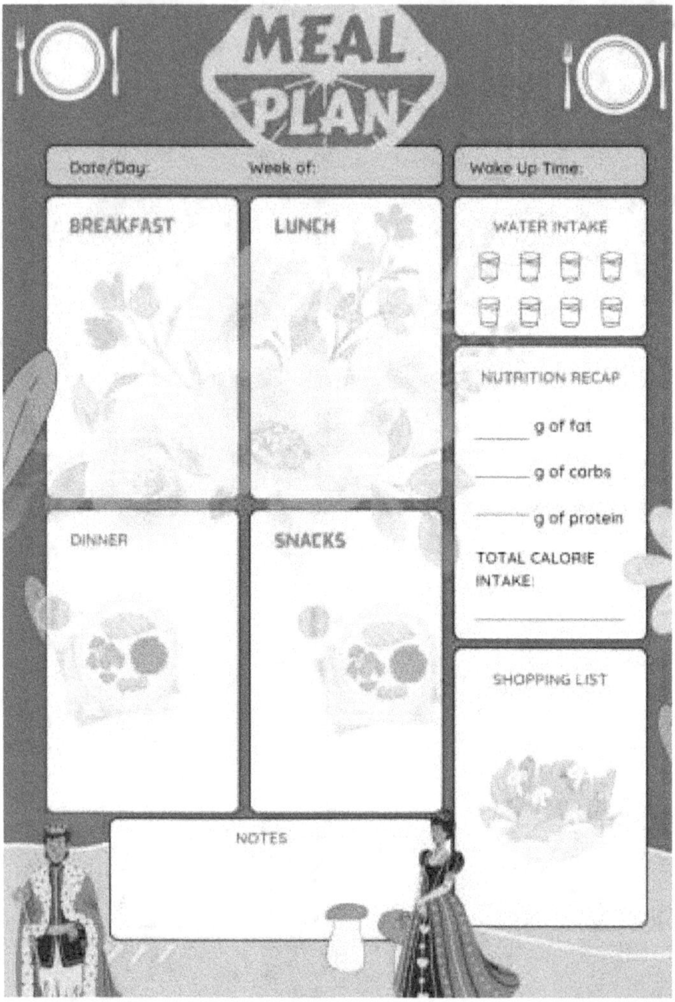

MEAL PLAN

| Date/Day: | Week of: | Wake Up Time: |

BREAKFAST

LUNCH

WATER INTAKE

DINNER

SNACKS

NUTRITION RECAP

_______ g of fat

_______ g of carbs

_______ g of protein

TOTAL CALORIE INTAKE:

____

SHOPPING LIST

NOTES

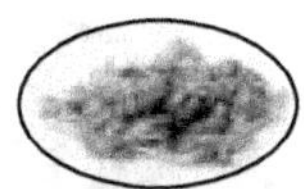
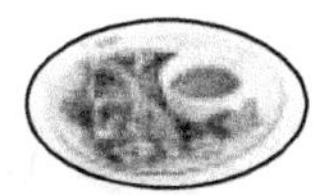
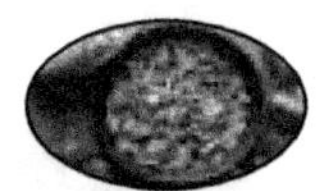

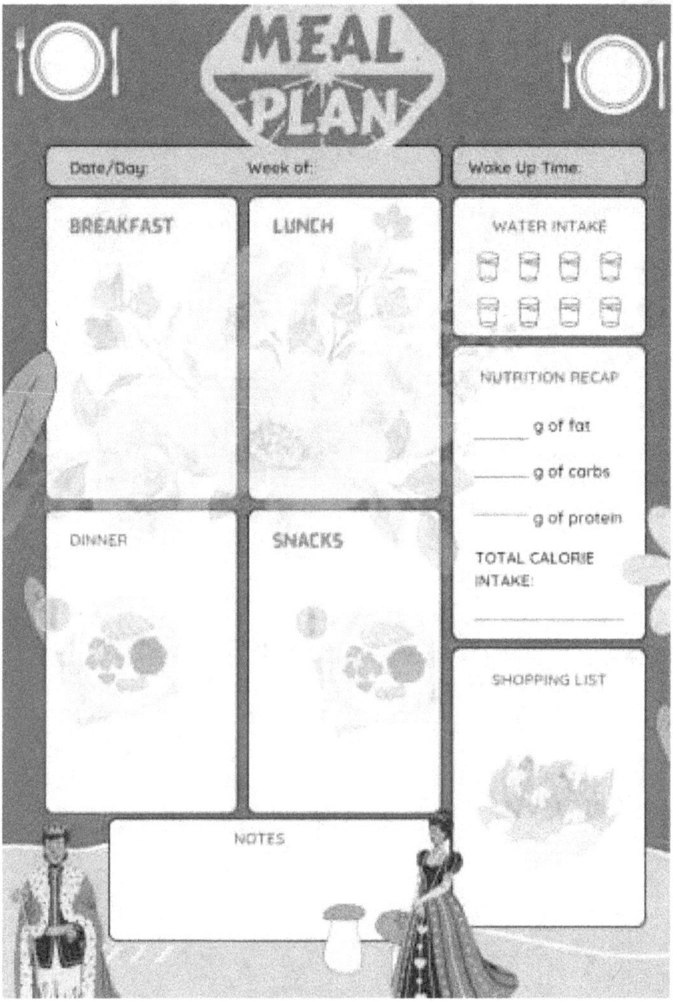

MEAL PLAN

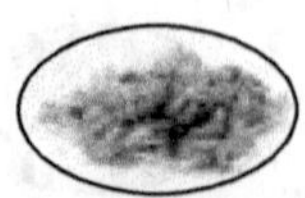
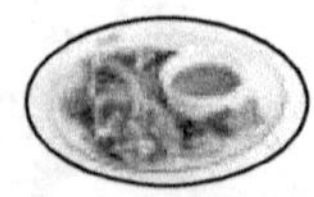
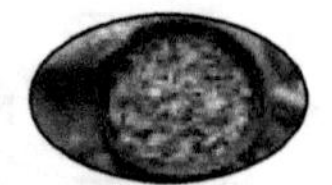

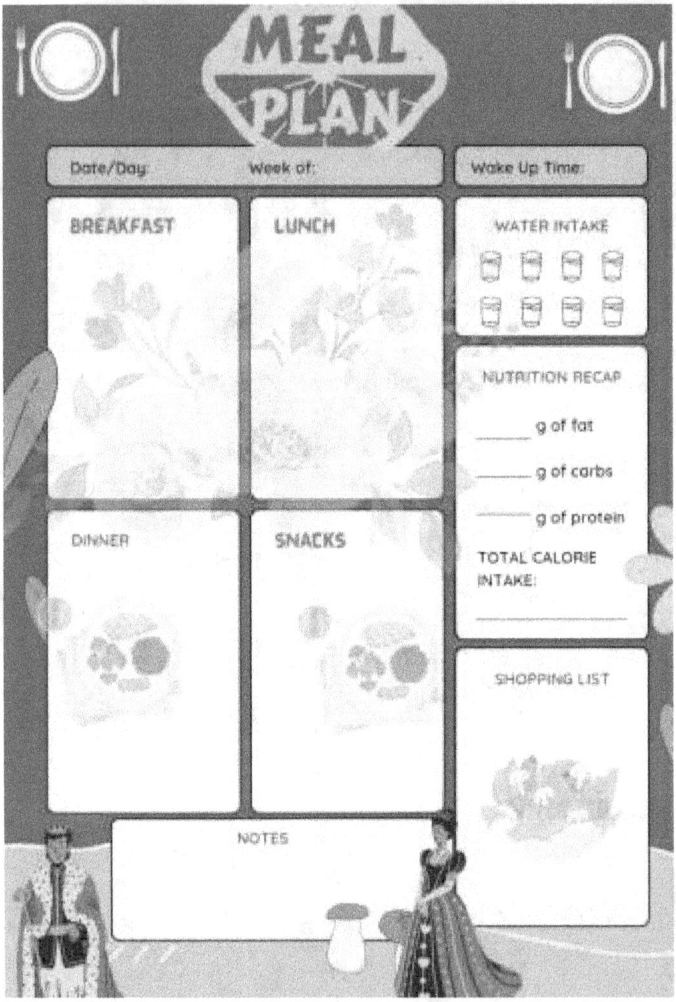

MEAL PLAN

| Date/Day: | Week of: | Wake Up Time: |

BREAKFAST

LUNCH

WATER INTAKE

NUTRITION RECAP

__________ g of fat

__________ g of carbs

__________ g of protein

TOTAL CALORIE INTAKE:

____

DINNER

SNACKS

SHOPPING LIST

NOTES

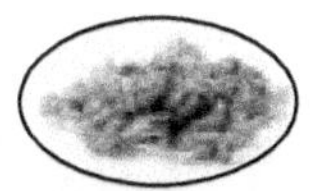 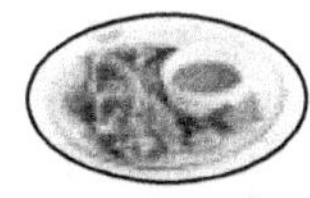 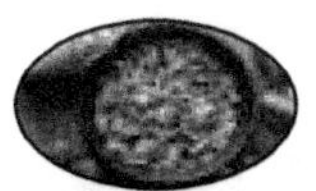

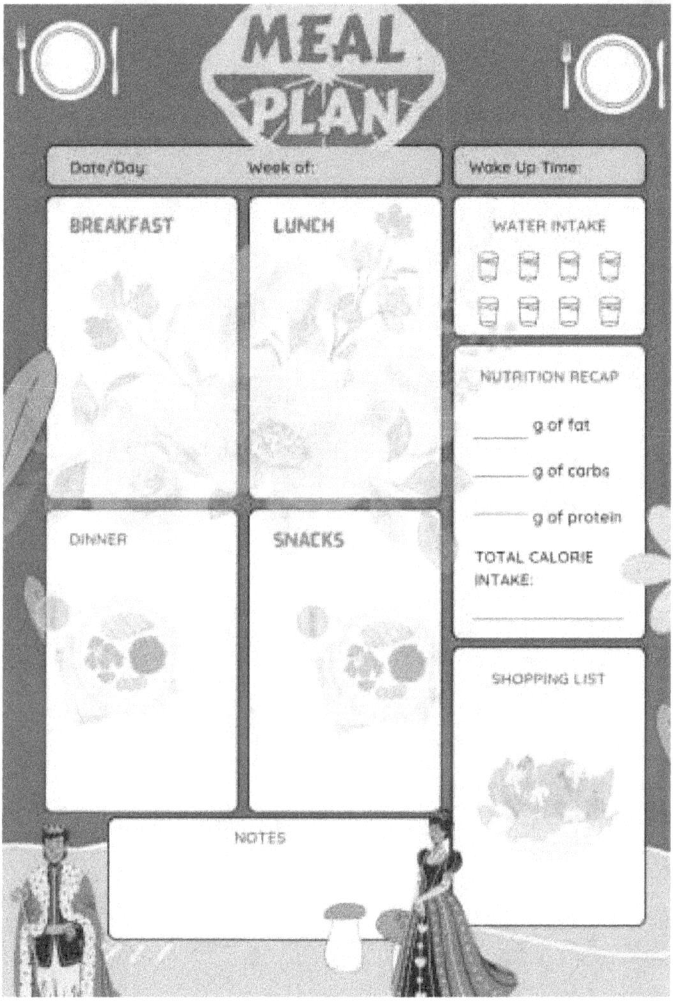

MEAL PLAN

| Date/Day | Week of: | Wake Up Time: |

BREAKFAST

LUNCH

WATER INTAKE

NUTRITION RECAP

__________ g of fat

__________ g of carbs

__________ g of protein

TOTAL CALORIE INTAKE:

____

DINNER

SNACKS

SHOPPING LIST

NOTES